Chronic
Pelvic Pain

Chronic Pelvic Pain

Edited by

Tin-Chiu Li MD PhD MRCP FRCOG

Professor of Reproductive Medicine and Surgery
Jessop Wing, Royal Hallamshire Hospital
Sheffield, UK

and

William L Ledger MA PhD FRCOG

Professor of Obstetrics and Gynaecology
Jessop Wing, Royal Hallamshire Hospital
Sheffield, UK

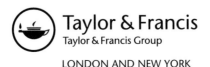

Taylor & Francis
Taylor & Francis Group

LONDON AND NEW YORK

© 2006 Taylor & Francis, an imprint of the Taylor & Francis Group

First published in the United Kingdom in 2006
by Taylor & Francis,
an imprint of the Taylor & Francis Group,
2 Park Square, Milton Park
Abingdon, Oxon OX14 4RN, UK

Tel.:   +44 (0) 20 7017 6000
Fax.:   +44 (0) 20 7017 6699
E-mail: info.medicine@tandf.co.uk
Website: http://www.tandf.co.uk/medicine

British Library Cataloguing in Publication Data

Data available on application

Library of Congress Cataloging-in-Publication Data

Data available on application

ISBN10: 0-415-38512-1
ISBN13: 9-78-0-415-38512-1

Distributed in North and South America by

Taylor & Francis
2000 NW Corporate Blvd
Boca Raton, FL 33431, USA

Within Continental USA
Tel.: 800 272 7737; Fax.: 800 374 3401
Outside Continental USA
Tel.: 561 994 0555; Fax.: 561 361 6018
E-mail: orders@crcpress.com

Distributed in the rest of the world by
Thomson Publishing Services
Cheriton House
North Way
Andover, Hampshire SP10 5BE, UK
Tel.: +44 (0) 1264 332424
E-mail: salesorder.tandf@thomsonpublishingservices.co.uk

Composition by Parthenon Publishing
Printed and bound by Antony Rowe Ltd., Chippenham, Wiltshire, UK

Contents

List of contributors

Ian Adam FRCS, Consultant Obstetrician and Gynaecologist, Royal Hallamshire Hospital, Sheffield, UK

Raya Al-Talib MB ChB FRCA, Associate Specialist in Anaesthesia, Shackleton Department of Anaesthetics, Southampton University Hospitals NHS Trust, Southampton, UK

Ying C Cheong MD MRCOG, Subspecialist Trainee in Reproductive Medicine, Jessop Wing, Royal Hallamshire Hospital, Sheffield, UK

Daniel J Fletcher MB BCh MRCS, Specialist Registrar, Royal Hallamshire Hospital, Sheffield, UK

Hany Lashen MB BCh PLAB MRCOG MD, Senior Lecturer in Obstetrics and Gynaecology, Jessop Wing, Royal Hallamshire Hospital, Sheffield, UK

William L Ledger MA PhD FRCOG, Professor of Obstetrics and Gynaecology, Academic Unit of Reproductive and Developmental Medicine, Jessop Wing, Royal Hallamshire Hospital, Sheffield, UK

Tin-Chiu Li MD PhD MRCP FRCOG, Professor of Reproductive Medicine and Surgery, Jessop Wing, Royal Hallamshire Hospital, Sheffield, UK

Soma Mukherjee MRCOG, Staff Grade in Obstetrics and Gynaecology, Heatherwood and Wexham Park Hospital, Slough, Berkshire, UK

Chun Ng MB ChB, Clinical Research Fellow in Reproductive Medicine, IVF Unit, Hammersmith Hospital, London, UK

Nick Plunkett FRCA FFPMANZCA, Consultant in Anaesthesia and Pain Management, Sheffield Training Hospitals, Sheffield, UK

Philip W Reginald MD FRCOG, Consultant Obstetrician and Gynaecologist, Heatherwood and Wexham Park Hospital, Slough, Berkshire, UK

Sheilagh Reid MB BCh BAO MD FRCS, Specialist Registrar, Department of Urology, Royal Hallamshire Hospital, Sheffield, UK

Mike Richmond FRCA, Consultant in Anaesthesia and Pain Management, Sheffield Training Hospitals, Sheffield, UK

Derek Rosario MB ChB FRCS MD, Consultant Urologist Surgeon, Royal Hallamshire Hospital, Sheffield, UK

Andrew J Shorthouse BSc MS FRCS, Consultant Surgeon and Honorary Senior Lecturer, Department of Colorectal Surgery, Northern General Hospital, Sheffield, UK

Pauline Slade BSc MSc PhD FBPsS CPsychol, Consultant Clinical Psychologist, Clinical Psychology Unit, Department of Psychology, University of Sheffield, Sheffield, UK

R William Stones MD FRCOG, Senior Lecturer in Obstetrics and Gynaecology, University of Southampton, Southampton, Hampshire, UK

Geoffrey Trew MB BS MRCOB, Consultant in Reproductive Medicine and Surgery, Hammersmith Hospital, London, UK

Alistair Warren BSc PhD, Senior Lecturer Biomedical Science, University of Sheffield, Sheffield, UK

Cornelia C T Wiesender MB BS MRCOG, Consultant Obstetrician and Gynaecologist, Department of Obstetrics and Gynaecology, Leicester General Hospital, Leicester, UK

Yat May Wong, Specialist in Obstetrics and Gynaecology, Kuala Lumpur, Malaysia

Preface

Chronic pelvic pain is a common and distressing condition in young women. Despite its high prevalence, chronic pelvic pain is poorly understood and difficult to manage. In many situations, the underlying cause is unclear, causing great frustration to patient and clinician. In others, pathology that is thought to be contributory may turn out to be coincidental. It is well recognized that treatment is often of limited success.

In May 2004, we arranged a national symposium on chronic pelvic pain in Sheffield with support from Shire Pharmaceuticals. Nationally prominent speakers with an interest in the condition were invited to contribute to the meeting. Following the meeting, we decided to publish the contributions of all the distinguished speakers in this book, *Chronic Pelvic Pain*, in order that we could share with our readers the experience of these various experts in the pathogenesis and management of this interesting condition. We hope that the work will help colleagues to manage these difficult and perplexing problems.

Tin-Chiu Li
William L Ledger

Foreword

The relief of pain and suffering has been the challenge of medicine from time immemorial; and despite the tremendous medical progress over the centuries, it remains a challenge.

Pain is a complex phenomenon; it is a symptom that may or may not be associated with obvious organic findings. Pain is subjective; in each case, the psychologic and organic aspects may be extremely difficult to separate. Therefore the patient's complaint of pain remains valid even if an organic cause cannot be identified. This is especially true for chronic pain, and indeed this is the reason why the definition of chronic pain is symptom-based rather than disease-based.

Chronic pelvic pain is a common disorder. It affects 15% of women of reproductive age. In the USA, 10% of all the outpatient gynecological consultations, are for chronic pelvic pain. The condition is associated with significant social costs due to decreased productivity, sick leave, medical costs, etc. In addition, the cost to the affected individual, in terms of pain, disability, psychological distress, and the effect of all of this on their partners and immediate family cannot be ignored.

Chronic pelvic pain may be cyclic and clearly related to the menstrual function; it may be related to physiological functions, such as micturition, defecation or sexual intercourse, or bear no temporal relationship to any of these. The temporal association may offer a clue to the cause of the pain. The causes of chronic pelvic pain may be gynecologic, intestinal, urologic, musculoskeletal, purely psychological or complemented by psychological factors. Not infrequently, as a result of the investigation, a cause for the pain will not be identified, or the presence of any lesion would simply be coincidental.

The preceding confirms the importance and the complexity of the condition; it underlines the necessity for physicians treating patients presenting with chronic pain to have special expertise in the field, and the need for a thorough clinical assessment and systematic investigation, complemented with a professional, patient, humane, positive and empathetic approach to the patient. Such an approach results in a good physician/health professional–patient relationship and rapport that are essential in the successful treatment of this condition.

It is therefore evident that chronic pain demands equal consideration of both organic and psychological factors. Proper initial clinical assessment, investigation and referral, as necessary, is more likely to lead to a correct diagnosis and management, and thus avoid the patient entering the vicious circle of interminable referrals and the associated, frequently unnecessary re-investigations. This also emphasizes the need for an early multidisciplinary approach to more complex cases and the value of special clinics in the successful management of such patients.

The book is well written, concise, and practical and reflects a multidisciplinary point of view. Yes, I have read all of its 14 chapters. It has a multidisciplinary authorship including specialists in gynecology, anesthesiology and pain management, urology, colorectal surgery, reproductive medicine and surgery, clinical psychology, and biomedical science. This text will be of great value to physicians and health professionals who care for patients with chronic pelvic pain.

Professor Victor Gomel
Department of Obstetrics and Gynecology
Faculty of Medicine
University of British Columbia
Vancouver BC, Canada

Basic pelvic neuroanatomy

Alistair Warren

INTRODUCTION

Chronic pelvic pain may be related to a large number of contributory factors, including: endometriosis, infections, adhesions, muscle pain, bone and joint pain, and many others[1]. On the premise that it is first necessary to understand the basic science that underpins any medical practice, this introductory chapter has three aims:

(1)   To provide an account of relevant female pelvic anatomy, with an emphasis on the nerve supply;

(2)   To outline some current concepts of visceral pain transmission; and

(3)   To note some clinical applications of the above.

SOME BASICS

Functionally, the nervous system may be divided into the somatic nervous system (SNS) and the autonomic nervous system (ANS). Strictly, the ANS consists of general visceral efferents, with visceral afferent fibers being classified separately (together the two comprise the visceral nervous system). However, it is considered useful here to include together both the sensory and the motor neurons that supply the viscera.

In the SNS, peripheral afferent nerves convey general somatic information (pain, touch, temperature and proprioception) from nerve endings in the skin, muscles and joints to the spinal cord. The cell bodies of these sensory nerves lie in dorsal root ganglia (DRG). Projections from the DRG pass into the spinal cord where they branch and pass up or down the cord, or go directly to the dorsal gray matter where they synapse with interneurons. These then synapse with large multipolar motor neurons (efferents) that lie in the ventral gray horn. Somatic motor neurons send axons to skeletal muscle through the ventral root. Anterior (ventral) primary rami branch and can communicate extensively with other rami via plexuses. Plexuses, such as the sacral plexus (made up of anterior primary rami of spinal segments L4 and 5, S1, 2 and 3), facilitate an overlap of the distribution of nerve supply by exchanging fibers between individual nerves, branches and fascicles.

Visceral afferent nerve fibers (which convey sensory information about the viscera) generally run with the visceral efferents of the ANS. The ANS is divided into two divisions: the sympathetic and the parasympathetic.

Sympathetic division

Sympathetic motor fibers originate from spinal levels T1–L2. Cell bodies of these preganglionic neurons lie in the intermediolateral cell columns (lateral horns of the gray matter) and run through the ventral root of the spinal cord along with somatic motor fibers. After a short distance these myelinated preganglionic fibers leave the anterior rami as the white rami communicantes and pass into the sympathetic chains. White rami communicantes are present only between T1 and L2. The sympathetic chains consist of about 22 ganglia that lie on each side of the spinal cord, lateral to the vertebral bodies. The chains extend from the cervical to the sacral regions and have relatively thick interganglionic connecting rami. They contain pre- and postganglionic efferents and afferent fibers. Since one preganglionic fiber can synapse with 15–20 postganglionic cells, its effects are spread widely throughout the body[2].

In the sympathetic chain, the preganglionic fibers can follow one of three paths:

(1) Synapse and leave the chain at the same level, as unmyelinated postganglionic sympathetic fibers, which often re-enter a spinal nerve through the grey rami communicantes. Gray rami are found on all spinal nerves;

(2) Pass up or down the sympathetic chain for a variable distance before synapsing and leaving the chain as above; or

(3) Pass through the chain without synapsing to form splanchnic nerves.

The greater (T5–10), lesser (T10–11), lowest (T12) and four lumbar splanchnic nerves (collectively known as the abdominopelvic splanchnic nerves) contain preganglionic sympathetic fibers that synapse in the prevertebral ganglia.

Prevertebral ganglia lie distal to the sympathetic chains. Cell bodies in these ganglia send postganglionic unmyelinated fibers to the abdominal and pelvic viscera (Table 1.1).

Postganglionic fibers form plexuses, the branches of which are distributed with arteries (see below). The nerves run between the tunica media and tunica adventitial layers of the vessels. Most postganglionic fibers are adrenergic, using noradrenaline as the neurotransmitter. However, those fibers that supply glands in the skin are cholinergic, using acetylcholine as their transmitter (but see later).

Afferents run from the viscera, with their efferent fibers, and convey information about visceral function as well as pain. Many of these afferents pass into the sympathetic chain where they can run up or down before passing through the white rami communicantes to reach the DRG, which, as with the somatic afferents, is the site of their cell body. The DRG neurons then project to the intermediolateral column of the spinal cord.

Parasympathetic division

The craniosacral outflow that makes up the parasympathetic division of the nervous system originates from:

(1)   Cranial nerves III, VII, IX and X;

(2)   Sacral roots 2, 3 and 4.

Only the sacral component is considered here, although in some ways its actions can be regarded simply as an extension of vagal functions.

Table 1.1   Prevertebral ganglia and viscera supplied

Prevertebral ganglion	Viscus supplied
Celiac	Liver, gallbladder, esophagus, stomach, pancreas, spleen, small intestine, suprarenal gland (fibers to the suprarenal gland, T8–L1, do not synapse in this ganglion but pass through to synapse in the adrenal medulla)
Superior mesenteric	Large intestine, rectum, internal anal sphincter
Inferior mesenteric	Bladder, kidney, gonads, clitoris

Parasympathetic motor fibers arise in gray matter at spinal levels S2, 3 and 4, and innervate the descending and sigmoid colon, rectum, pelvic viscera and erectile tissues of the external genitalia. Apart from at the external genitalia, parasympathetic fibers do not reach the body wall and generally do not run in spinal nerves (except in proximal parts of the anterior rami of spinal segments S2, 3 and 4). The long myelinated preganglionic fibers synapse at small parasympathetic ganglia located close to, or often within, the viscus they supply. The postganglionic parasympathetic fibers are therefore short and unmyelinated; they are cholinergic.

For both parasympathetic and sympathetic divisions the neurotransmitter between pre- and postganglionic fibers is acetylcholine. However, it is now recognized that there are many neurotransmitters and cotransmitters in the autonomic nervous system, as well as elsewhere[3]. For example, non-adrenergic, non-cholinergic (NANC) nerves are functionally very important and include nerves with neurotransmitters such as purines, peptides, nitric oxide and many others (see below).

In most parts of the body, parasympathetic fibers are concerned with the transmission of physiological information about normal visceral function, while visceral pain is signaled through sympathetic fibers. However, pelvic parasympathetic afferent fibers also conduct pain. They have their nerve cell body in the DRG of spinal segments S2, 3 and 4.

NERVE SUPPLY OF THE PELVIS – AN OUTLINE

Somatic innervation of the pelvis is supplied by the sacral plexus. It lies on the posterior wall of the lesser pelvis, close to the piriformis muscle, and receives nerve roots from lumbar and sacral segments L4–S3. Branches from the roots supply the levator ani (see below), piriformis (S1, 2) and coccygeus (S3, 4) muscles.

Autonomic sympathetic innervation comes from spinal segments T10–L2, which travel with spinal nerves and blood vessels to their targets. Parasympathetic supply comes from the pelvic splanchnic nerves (nervi erigentes), derived from sacral segments S2, 3 and 4. These contain both efferent and afferent preganglionic parasympathetic nerves. The efferents cause relaxation of the internal anal and internal urinary sphincters when their organs contract, and the afferents are sensory to them. The efferents also cause dilatation of blood vessels in the erectile tissues resulting in tumescence of the clitoris and erection in the penis.

NERVE SUPPLY OF THE PELVIS – SOMATIC SUPPLY

The pudendal nerve arises from the anterior divisions of the ventral rami of sacral segments S2, 3 and 4. It remains retroperitoneal and supplies the external genitalia and the perineum. Initially, the nerve leaves the pelvis through the greater sciatic foramen, between the piriformis and coccygeus muscles, then nips back into the pelvis through the lesser sciatic foramen where it runs in the lateral part of the ischiorectal fossa to reach perineum. Here it provides somatic motor supply to the superficial perineal muscles. At least part of the motor supply to the pubococcygeus muscle may come from the perineal branches of the pudendal nerve, as does the sensory supply to the lower vagina (the upper vagina lacks somatic innervation). The inferior hemorrhoidal branches of the pudendal nerve, along with nerves from the middle and superior rectal plexuses, supply the anus and rectum. The inferior hemorrhoidal nerves are motor to the striated external urethral and external anal sphincters and sensory to the lower and middle third of the anal canal, parts of the upper third[4] and skin of the labia and perianal region. The pudendal nerve terminates distally as the purely afferent dorsal nerve of the clitoris. It may be located easily for pudendal nerve block where it hooks around the ischial spine, just lateral to the attachment of the sacrospinous ligament. A pudendal nerve block anesthetizes, amongst other things, the genitalia and external urethral sphincter but not the internal urethral sphincter; this is supplied by fibers directly from the sacral plexus and therefore maintains urinary continence.

A small perineal branch of spinal segment S4 supplies the external anal sphincter and surrounding skin, with the perforating (cutaneous) branch of S2 and 3 supplying the gluteal skin. The tiny coccygeal plexus (S4, 5, Co 1) supplies a patch of skin from the coccyx to the anus and, more importantly, part of the levator ani, the coccygeus muscle and the sacrococcygeal joint.

The obturator nerve runs along the lateral wall of the pelvis on its journey from the lumbar plexus (lumbar segments L2, 3 and 4) to supply the medial muscles of the thigh. It passes out of the pelvis via the obturator canal where it divides into anterior and posterior branches. Damage to this nerve (e.g. from compression by the fetal head) may affect the medial adductor muscles of the lower limb as well as its sensory area (medial thigh, occasionally as far as the medial side of the knee).

NERVE SUPPLY OF THE PELVIS – AUTONOMIC SUPPLY

The sympathetic innervation of the lower limb, and of the inferior hypogastric plexus, comes from the sacral sympathetic ganglia, which represent the inferior termination of the sympathetic chains. Gray rami communicantes from the sacral sympathetic ganglia take postganglionic sympathetic fibers to each of the sacral and coccygeal anterior rami, enabling them to contribute to the sacral plexus and thereby supply sympathetic fibers to the lower limbs. The chains eventually fuse in the midline, over the coccyx, to give the ganglion impar. This small and relatively unimportant structure is effectively the coccygeal ganglion. Some segmental sympathetic supplies are shown in Table 1.2[2].

The celiac plexus is the largest of the autonomic plexuses in the body. It lies close to the celiac arterial trunk and consists of the two celiac ganglia connected by a network of nerve fibers. The vagus cranial nerves and phrenic nerves also contribute, along with the greater and lesser splanchnic nerves. A number of lesser plexuses can be identified, either as subdivisions of the main plexus or as secondary plexuses that follow arteries nearby. Of particular relevance to the pelvis are the hypogastric plexuses.

The superior hypogastric plexus (sometimes called the presacral nerve) lies between the common iliac arteries, anterior to the body of the fifth lumbar

Table 1.2 Segmental sympathetic supplies

Organ	Spinal supply
Kidney	T10–L1
Ureter	T11–L2
Suprarenal gland	T8–L1
Gonads	T10–T11
Urinary bladder	T11–L2
Uterus	T12–L1
Uterine tube	T10–L1

vertebra and sacral promontory, and comprises branches of the aortic plexus and third and fourth lumbar splanchnic nerves. It supplies the ureteric, ovarian and common iliac plexuses and contains sympathetic fibers. A few parasympathetics may also join via the inferior hypogastric plexus (from the pelvic splanchnic nerves), or they may run independently to supply the sigmoid and descending colon, the left colic flexure and the left part of the transverse colon. The superior hypogastric plexus divides into two 'nerves' that join the inferior hypogastric plexus. The inferior hypogastric or pelvic plexus lies in extraperitoneal connective tissue anterior to the sacral and coccygeal plexuses, lateral to the cervix and rectum, and medial to the levator ani and the internal iliac arteries. There are many small ganglia distributed throughout the plexus and these may supply some sympathetic branches, although most come from the hypogastric nerves. Parasympathetic fibers come from the pelvic splanchnic nerves.

The uterovaginal plexus is the part of the inferior hypogastric plexus that lies in the broad ligament. Sympathetic fibers run from this plexus to the uterus to provide 'a motor facilitating function in relation to the smooth muscle fibers of the uterus'[4]. They probably also supply afferent fibers to determine stretch from the uterus, uterine tubes and the broad ligament. Parasympathetic fibers in the pelvic splanchnics (from sacral segments S2, 3 and 4) synapse in the paracervical ganglion (within a small plexus of nerves that come from the uterovaginal plexus) to supply the uterus. Although predominantly influenced by hormones, in the uterus parasympathetic activity may produce vasodilatation and inhibition of uterine smooth muscle contraction, while a sympathetic stimulus causes the opposite effect[2]. Pain from the uterus is often referred to areas supplied by the sacral nerves and spinal segment T12; that is, the lower back and inferior hypogastrum. Uterine spasm and salpingitis may cause pain referred to the back, pubic, inguinal and anterior thigh areas (i.e. dermatomes T12–L2).

The uterine tubes receive sympathetic innervation from spinal segments T10–L1 via the hypogastric plexus. The ovaries probably receive their sympathetic supply from segments T10 and 11, via the ovarian and uterine plexuses, which travel with the ovarian artery. Parasympathetic supply of the tubes derives from two sources:

(1)   Medial parts of the tube are innervated from pelvic splanchnics; and

(2)   Lateral parts (and the ovaries) are supplied by the vagus cranial nerve[5].

Rogers comments that while sympathetic fibers supply the smooth muscle of blood vessels in the uterine tubes, parasympathetic fibers supply the smooth muscle of the tubal wall[5]. Fibers from the inferior hypogastric and uterovaginal plexuses also supply the walls of the vagina, the clitoris and the vestibular glands. They are generally parasympathetic and cause vasodilatation.

The ureters are supplied from several nearby plexuses, including the hypogastric. Afferents run back to spinal segments T11–L2 and pain is usually referred to the groin. The vesical nerve plexus, from the anterior parts of the hypogastric plexus, supplies the bladder. It is made up of sympathetics (from spinal segments T11–L2) and parasympathetics from the pelvic splanchnic nerves. Parasympathetic efferents are motor to the detrusor muscle and inhibitory to the internal sphincter muscles. Afferents detect stretch in the bladder and act reflexively to contract the bladder muscle and relax the sphincter. Pain from the inferior part of the bladder takes the parasympathetic route while that from the superior part follows sympathetics to T11–L2.

THE BONY PELVIS

Although continuous inferiorly with the abdominal cavity, the adult pelvic cavity is directed posteriorly so that the plane of the bony pelvic inlet lies at about 55° to the horizontal. The pelvic inlet (or brim) separates the greater and lesser pelvis. The inlet is bounded by the upper line of the pubic symphysis, pubic crest and tubercle, pectineal line, iliopubic eminence, arcuate line of the ilium, ala of the sacrum and the sacral promontory. Inferiorly the borders of the bony pelvic outlet consist of the lower line of the pubic symphysis, the ischial tuberosities and the lower part of the sacrum and coccyx. Additionally, a number of ligaments contribute posteriorly to the pelvic basin, including the sacrotuberous, sacrospinous, sacroiliac (anterior and posterior) and sacrococcygeal (anterior and posterior) ligaments. The paired ilium, pubic and ischium bones, along with the single sacrum (including the coccyx), make up the bony pelvis. The hip joint includes the head of the femur and the acetabulum of the hip (innominate) bone. It is supplied by the femoral nerve (and its muscular branches), the obturator nerve, the superior gluteal nerves and branches of the nerves to the quadratus femoris muscle[6].

WALLS AND FLOOR OF THE PELVIS

The anterior (which is also inferior), posterior (also superior) and lateral walls are essentially bony. Anteriorly lies the pubic symphysis, body and rami while posteriorly the sacrum, coccyx, sacroiliac joints and medial aspects of the iliac bones and ligaments make up the walls. The hip bones constitute the bulk of the lateral wall. The large obturator foramen is closed by both fascia (of the obturator membrane) and the obturator internus muscle, which is supplied by its own nerve from spinal segments L5, S1 and S2. Obturator internus leaves the lesser pelvis via the lesser sciatic foramen to attach to the greater trochanter of the femur. Immediately anterior to this attachment lies the insertion of piriformis muscle, which leaves the lesser pelvis via the greater sciatic foramen. Piriformis originates over the sacrum, the upper part of the sciatic notch and the sacrotuberous ligament. It is supplied by the ventral rami of sacral nerves S1 and S2. The sacral plexus lies between piriformis posteriorly and the internal iliac vessels and ureters anteriorly. The sacral anterior primary rami lie behind the thin fascial covering of piriformis and are covered by this fascia as it joins the sacral periosteum[7].

The pelvic floor is a muscular funnel also known as the pelvic diaphragm. It consists largely of the levator ani and coccygeus muscles sandwiched between their superior and inferior fascial coverings. The coccygeus (also called ischiococcygeus) is a small, variable, triangular sheet of muscle that arises from the ischial spine and blends with the sacrospinous ligament. Posteriorly it attaches to the fifth sacral segment and lateral parts of the coccyx. The coccygeus is supplied by spinal segments S3 and S4 and, unlike in some quadrupeds where it helps to 'wag the tail', in humans it acts largely with the levator ani.

The levator ani is a large muscle of variable thickness that, with its pair, forms the bulk of the pelvic floor. It attaches to the pelvic surface of the body of the pubic bone anteriorly and to the ischial spine laterally. Between these bony attachments it joins the long tendonous arch, or thickening, of the fascia over the obturator internus muscle. The two levator ani muscles run medially to insert together into several midline structures: the perineal body, the anal canal, the anococcygeal ligament and the coccyx. Physiologically it is described as a predominately slow-twitch muscle[8]. Its fibers may be subdivided into a number of named groups.

The pubococcygeus arises from the back of the pubic body and arch anteriorly, and from the tendonous arch laterally, to run posteriorly to insert into the coccyx and anococcygeal raphe. Some fibers run to the wall of the vagina (as the pubovaginalis muscle) while others run medially to surround the urethra (sphincter urethrae). Further back, other fibers run into the perineal body and rectum (as the puboanalis). This muscle forms the conjoint coat by blending with longitudinal muscles of the rectum and their overlying fascia. Some lower fibers of the puboanalis run behind the anorectal junction inferiorly and cross over to meet those from the opposite side to form the puborectal sling. This sling also incorporates fibers from the external anal sphincter. A few aponeurotic fibers run from the obturator fascia to the lower part of the coccyx (called iliococcygeus, which also forms part of the anococcygeal ligament). Usually the lateral pubococcygeal fibers lie superior to the anterior iliococcygeal fibers. The iliococcygeus muscle has a small posterior slip called the iliosacralis.

Sacral roots S2 and S3 supply most of the levator ani. In summary, the pudendal nerve supplies the anteromedial part and direct branches from the sacral plexus supply the remainder. Wendell Smith and Wilson have reported the various pathways by which fibers from these sacral roots reach the pelvic floor and perineal muscles[8]. Fibers from typical motoneurons close to Onuf's nucleus leave the spinal cord through S2 and 3 nerve roots to innervate the pelvic floor muscles from above and the perineal muscles (via the inferior hemorrhoidal nerves, branches of the anococcygeal nerves or the perineal branch of S4) from below. The anterior part of the levator ani (and sphincter urethrae) receive their somatic motor innervation in a variety of ways, including: the pelvic splanchnic nerves (where somatic motor fibers run with autonomic fibers); through a separate nerve from the sacral plexus; or in a branch of the pudendal nerve that originates above the ischial spine. Somatic motor fibers to the posterior part of the levator ani and puboanalis appear to travel by one of three routes: with autonomic fibers from the inferior hypogastric plexus; in branches off those supplying the anterior part of the levator ani; or directly from the sacral plexus.

The perineal muscles can be contracted voluntarily, but are also 'functionally coupled with viscera'[8]. Their nerve supply originates in the ventral horn of sacral segments S2 and 3, from a group of atypical motoneurons that lie in Onuf's nucleus X[9].

SOME CURRENT CONCEPTS IN VISCERAL PAIN TRANSMISSION

Since the perception of pain can vary so dramatically depending on circumstances it is no surprise that the mechanisms involved in nociception are likely to be complex. There are many descriptions in the literature of nociception, nociceptive receptors and pathways, and the management of pain (e.g. Hawthorn and Redmond[10]). The following is a brief account of current concepts in the study of visceral pain.

Most studies of pain mechanisms are based on experimental models of somatic pain, not visceral pain. The implication is that all pain has a similar neurobiological mechanism. Recently, however, this approach has been questioned as there are important differences, as well as similarities, between observations on the mechanisms of visceral and somatic pain.

Five clinical characteristics of visceral pain have been identified[11]:

(1) It does not occur in all viscera (especially not solid organs such as the liver);

(2) It is not always the result of trauma;

(3) Typically it is poorly localized;

(4) It is often referred elsewhere; and

(5) It often occurs with autonomic reflexes, including nausea etc.

Previously, two opposing views on visceral pain existed. In essence these were:

(1) That viscera are innervated by different types of receptors for different stimuli, for example receptors for homeostatic regulation or for sensory perception (including pain) – this is analogous to somatic nociception; and

(2) That viscera have a single receptor type that works at low levels of stimulation to provide normal regulatory information, while at high frequency of activation it can signal pain.

However, there is now evidence for two separate classes of nociceptor in viscera[12]. Firstly, there are receptors with a high threshold to physiological stimuli. These are activated only by stimuli that would be described as noxious (that is, in the noxious range). Such receptors have been reported in the uterus, the urinary bladder and other pelvic organs. Secondly, there are receptors with a low threshold to physiological stimuli that can be activated across a wide range, from mild (innocuous) to intense (noxious) stimuli. These receptors can signal the intensity of the stimulus in their firing pattern (known as intensity-encoding receptors).

Another consideration is that many visceral afferents only become activated at a level that can be perceived when the tissue they supply is inflamed[11]. These receptors are normally unresponsive and only become sensitized to respond in the presence of chemical mediators such as 5-hydroxytryptamine[13]. These 'silent' receptors are concerned with tissue inflammation rather than mechanical stimuli such as distension. However, some authors believe that the clinical value of these silent nociceptors and their role in visceral pain '…remains to be established'[11]. Their hypothesis for visceral pain involves instead the two receptor classes described earlier. In this model, acute visceral pain activates high-threshold afferents. Chronic stimulation (such as inflammation or ischemia) causes sensitization of the high-threshold receptors. These sensitized nociceptors can now respond to previously innocent stimuli that form part of normal visceral activity. Such stimulation will persist until the sensitization ceases. Furthermore, the inflammation will affect normal visceral function, a change that may itself sensitize other nociceptors, thereby exacerbating the overall effect. Consequently, the effect of the initial injury may persist for some time, and indeed be greater after the acute damage has been repaired than it was at the time of injury. Repetitive stimulation from visceral afferent fibers increases the excitability of viscerosomatic neurons in the spinal cord[14]. In somatic nociception such sensitivity is coincident with a frequency-dependent increase in neuronal excitability (known as 'wind-up'). However, in visceral transmission the increased sensitivity does not appear to be due to wind-up but may be related to neurotransmitters and feedback effects within neural networks[11].

As mentioned above, the traditional view that the ANS contains only cholinergic and adrenergic neurotransmitters is now known to be a great oversimplification. Nerve terminals may contain several transmitter substances that not only co-localize in the presynaptic terminal, but are genuine cotransmitters[3]. Adenosine triphosphate (ATP) appears to be a very common cotransmitter that occurs with more established neurotransmitters in many parts of the nervous system. It causes excitatory junction potentials in sympathetic nerve stimulation of visceral smooth muscle, while noradrenaline activates second messenger systems that have little effect on the membrane potential[3].

The functional significance of cotransmission lies in the flexibility it generates beyond the 'all or none' action potential. Single action potentials can stimulate the release of small molecules of neurotransmitters, while trains of impulses are required to cause the release of larger neuropeptide transmitters. In the autonomic nervous system, ATP is released at low-frequency stimulation, while high frequencies favor noradrenaline and acetylcholine release. Multiple transmitters can act at different postsynaptic targets. When this is combined with possibilities of mixed excitatory and inhibitory effects from different cotransmitters, and presynaptic modulation (where a cotransmitter feeds back on presynaptic receptors that modulate its own, or another cotransmitter's, release), the possibilities for elaborate control of neural transmission become enormous. As Burnstock[3] recommends, the classification of nerves as 'adrenergic', 'peptidergic', 'nitrergic', etc. should be abandoned, although the descriptive terms of adrenergic, peptidergic and nitrergic transmission remain useful.

CONCLUSION

There remains a great deal to learn about the detection and transmission of chronic visceral pain. However, advances in molecular and developmental biology, and in anatomical imaging techniques (e.g. Venuti et al.[15]), continue to provide new insights into the basic scientific mechanisms that are essential to inform clinical practice.

REFERENCES

1.   Moore J, Kennedy S. Causes of chronic pelvic pain. Bailliere's Best Pract Res Clin Obstet Gynaecol 2000; 14: 389–402.

2.   Berry M, Bannister LH, Standring SM. Nervous system. In Williams PL, Bannister LH, Berry M, et al., eds. Gray's Anatomy: the Anatomical Basis of Medicine and Surgery, 38th edn. New York: Churchill Livingstone, 1995: 1293.

3.   Burnstock G. Cotransmission. Curr Opin Pharmacol 2004; 4: 47–52.

4.   Swash M. Neurology and neurophysiology of the female genital organs. In Phillipp E, Setchell M, Ginsburg J, eds. Scientific Foundations of Obstetrics and Gynaecology, 4th edn. Oxford: Butterworth-Heinemann, 1991: 110–11.

5.   Rogers AW. Textbook of Anatomy. Edinburgh: Churchill Livingstone, 1992: 657–73.

6. Soames RW. Skeletal system. In Williams PL, Bannister LH, Berry MM, et al., eds. Gray's Anatomy: the Anatomical Basis of Medicine and Surgery, 38th edn. New York: Churchill Livingstone, 1995: 685–7.

7. Salmons S. Muscle. In Williams PL, Bannister LH, Berry MM, et al., eds. Gray's Anatomy: the Anatomical Basis of Medicine and Surgery, 38th. New York: Churchill Livingstone, 1995: 830.

8. Wendell Smith CP, Wilson PM. The vulva, vagina and urethra and the musculature of the pelvic floor. In Phillipp E, Setchell M, Ginsburg J, et al., eds. Scientific Foundations of Obstetrics and Gynaecology, 4th edn. Oxford: Butterworth-Heinemann, 1991: 96–7.

9. Schroder HD. Onuf's nucleus X: a morphological study of a human spinal nucleus. Anat Embryol (Berl) 1981; 162: 443–53.

10. Hawthorn J, Redmond K. Pain: Causes and Management. Oxford: Blackwell Books, 1999.

11. Cervero F, Laird JMA. Visceral Pain. Lancet 1999; 353: 2145–8.

12. Cervero F. Sensory innervation of the viscera: peripheral basis of visceral pain. Physiol Rev 1994; 74: 95–138.

13. Heppelmann B, Messlinger K, Schaible H-G, Schmidt RF. Nociception and pain. Curr Opin Neurobiol 1991; 1: 192–7.

14. Roza C, Laird JMA, Cervero F. Spinal mechanisms underlying persistent pain and referred hyperalgesia in rats with an experimental ureteric stone. J Neurophysiol 1998; 79: 1603–12.

15. Venuti JM, Imielinska C, Molholt P. New views of male pelvic anatomy: role of computer-generated 3D images 1. Clin Anat 2004; 17: 261–71.

2

Common causes and protocol for investigation of chronic pelvic pain

Chun Ng, Geoffrey Trew

INTRODUCTION

Aristotle defined pain as 'the passion of the soul', but a more useful definition by the International Association for the Study of Pain is as 'an unpleasant sensory or emotional experience associated with actual or potential tissue damage, or described in terms of such damage'[1]. The experience of pain will always be subjective and will be affected by factors in the sufferer's environment, both physical and psychological. The definition of pain avoids tying pain to the stimulus[2]. In the assessment of patients with chronic pain, it is useful to be able to use an objective, clear and widely acknowledged definition for the condition of interest so that no ambiguity exists between clinicians in deciding treatment. Unfortunately, there is no such internationally agreed consensus on the definition of chronic pelvic pain. Most, but not all, authors have used a duration of 6 or more months as the major criterion for the definition of chronicity. Chronic pelvic pain has been described by Howard[2] as 'non-cyclic pain of 6 or more months' duration that localizes to the anatomic pelvis, anterior abdominal wall at or below the umbilicus, the lumbosacral back, or the buttocks, and is of sufficient severity as to cause functional disability or lead to medical care'. The prevalence of chronic pelvic pain in the general population appears to be high, and remarkably little is known about its pathophysiology. In the UK, chronic pelvic pain is estimated to have an annual incidence of 3.8% in women aged 15–73 years, which is higher than the figure reported for migraine (2.1%) and comparable to those for asthma (3.7%) and back pain (4.1%)[3].

The etiology of chronic pelvic pain is often not obvious. Traditionally, chronic pelvic pain has been managed by gynecologists, and this may have led to a narrow view of the possible causes. Every structure in the abdomen and/or pelvis could have a role in the etiology of chronic pelvic pain. Therefore, it is essential to think beyond the organs of the upper reproductive tract and also consider contributions from the peripheral and central nervous system, blood vessels, muscles and fascia of the abdominal wall and pelvic floor, gastrointestinal system and urological organs. Very occasionally, a disorder of only one of these is the cause, and treatment is curative. However, the pain is more often associated with several causes, and a number of contributing factors need to be evaluated and treated. Part of the dilemma in the evaluation of chronic pelvic pain is the assumption that pain can be linked with some form of pathology or obvious tissue damage[4]. Complex interactions occur among the reproductive organs, urinary tract and gastrointestinal system. Psychological and behavioral factors are known to contribute to the pain experience. The prevalence of major depression is elevated among patients with chronic pain, with estimates of 30–45%, compared with 5–17% in the general population. Personality disorders have a significant impact on behavioral responses to pain, and are negative predictors for response to therapy and return to normal functionality[5].

COMMON CAUSES OF CHRONIC PELVIC PAIN

There are many disorders that may be associated with chronic pelvic pain; a list of possible disorders is given in Table 2.1. This list is by no means exhaustive. The more common or major causes of chronic pelvic pain encountered in the UK will be described in more detail.

Endometriosis

Endometriosis is the presence of endometrial glands or stroma outside the uterine cavity. Endometriosis is a common cause of chronic pelvic pain. Currently, no valid epidemiological data exist to establish the true incidence of endometriosis in women with chronic pelvic pain. However, estimates of the percentage of women with chronic pelvic pain who also have endometriosis are as high as 70–90%[6]. The chronology of the development of pain due to endometriosis can be highly variable. The typical history of endometriosis starts with significant dysmenorrhea during adolescence, which may become progressively more severe with time. As endometriosis develops, the duration of menstrual cramps becomes longer and the cramps more severe. With the passage of time, premenstrual pain then ensues, with the duration and severity of pain gradually increasing until the person may have pain on an essentially continuous basis. Even when this pattern has become established, premenstrual and menstrual exacerbation of the pain often remains superimposed on the more continuous discomforts. Central deep

Table 2.1 Disorders that may be associated with chronic pelvic pain

Gynecological	*Musculoskeletal*
Adenomyosis	Chronic coccygeal pain
Adhesions	Compression of lumbar vertebrae
Adnexal mass	Degenerative joint disease
Cervical stenosis	Disc prolapse
Chronic endometritis	Fibromyositis
Endometrial or cervical polyps	Hernias
Endometriosis	Lumbar lordosis from pregnancy
Endosalpingiosis	Malignancy
Fibroids	Muscle strains or sprains
Herpes	Myofascial pains
Intrauterine contraceptive device	Nerve entrapment
Malignancy	Neuralgia
Ovarian remnant syndrome	Piriformis syndrome
Ovulatory pain	Referred pain
Pelvic congestive syndrome	Spondylosis
Pelvic inflammatory disease	
Residual accessory ovary	*Gastrointestinal*
Trapped ovary syndrome	Chronic constipation
Vulvodynia	Colitis
	Diverticulitis
Urological	Hernias
Chronic urinary tract infection	Inflammatory bowel disease
Chronic urethral syndrome	Irritable bowel syndrome
Interstitial cystitis	Malignancy
Malignancy	
Radiation cystitis	*Others*
Recurrent urethritis/cystitis	Depression
Renal stones	Personality disorder
Urethral carbuncle	Neurologic dysfunction
Urethral diverticulum	Porphyria
	Sleep disturbances

dyspareunia will often be present as well. Predictably, this is first noticed around the time of menstruation and then gradually becomes present throughout the remainder of the menstrual month[7].

The link between endometriosis and pain is not straightforward. Some women with laparoscopic evidence of endometriosis have no pain at all[8]. Between 2 and 43% of asymptomatic women are found to have endometriosis[9]. The discrepancies may have multiple explanations. The earlier, more inflammatory forms probably cause more pain than the 'burnt out' forms. This superficial form of the disease may cause pain by releasing inflammatory mediators of pain, such as bradykinins and prostaglandins. Nodular disease and endometriomas are distinct disease entities that develop and behave quite differently to superficial peritoneal disease[10]. Extensive nodular disease in the rectovaginal space may appear at laparoscopy as a few blue or black pin pricks on the uterosacral ligaments. Pain associated with these forms of endometriosis may be caused by traction on tissues, or by infiltration or constriction of nerves[11].

Physical examination findings include a nodular sensation in the pouch of Douglas and along the uterosacral ligaments. However, this is often a late finding and it is difficult to ascertain with certainty during pelvic examination. More commonly, the pouch of Douglas and the uterosacral ligaments are simply tender during examination, replicating the pain of deep dyspareunia[7]. Similarly, endometrial implants around the ovaries and on the broad ligaments almost always cannot be felt, although the areas of tenderness frequently correspond to the areas of endometriosis when seen at laparoscopy.

Pelvic congestion syndrome

This syndrome is typically a condition of the reproductive years and, in contrast to endometriosis, is equally prevalent among parous and nulliparous women[12]. Pelvic congestion syndrome is a clinical syndrome based on the characteristic symptom complex described by Beard and colleagues[13]. Pelvic congestion presents as an aching pain interspersed with acute episodes of sharp pain. It often starts as premenstrual ache with or without mid-cycle pain (mittelschmerz), which in time may spread through the whole cycle. Typically, the pain occurs predominantly on one side of the lower abdomen or the other but, unlike the pain of endometriosis, will always have occurred occasionally on the other side. The pain is brought on or exacerbated by prolonged standing, exercise or following a bowel motion. Severity is related to the stage of the menstrual cycle, and is worst in the second half. A unique symptom of pelvic congestion syndrome is postcoital ache, which must be distinguished from dyspareunia occurring at the time of coitus. This may persist for up to 48 hours after intercourse[14].

Physical examination for pelvic congestion can reveal suggestive, but not conclusive, findings. The findings on clinical examination are typically pain on deep palpation in the adnexae, with one side being more severe than the other; a bluish discoloration of the vagina; excess of a white, non-infective vaginal discharge;

and pelvic tenderness, particularly over one or both of the ovaries, less so on palpation of the uterus[14]. Radiological features of pelvic congestion are dilated uterine and ovarian veins with reduced venous clearance of contrast medium. The observation of ovarian vein reflux during transuterine venography is not a necessary condition for the diagnosis. The scoring system used for transuterine venograms includes as variables the diameter of the ovarian veins, the distribution of vessels, and the delay in clearance of contrast medium. Dilated pelvic veins can also be seen using transabdominal or transvaginal ultrasonography. However, the use of ultrasound to replace venography is controversial, especially because reflux at the origin of the ovarian vein is difficult to visualize and flow rates are low, making it difficult to obtain a satisfactory spectral display using Doppler. Thus, the venous clearance element of pelvic congestion, well seen using transuterine venography, is difficult to reproduce[12].

Adhesions

Pelvic adhesions can be caused by pelvic inflammatory disease, endometriosis, appendicitis, previous abdominal surgery or inflammatory bowel disease. Adhesions are diagnosed in about 25% of women with chronic pelvic pain[15]. The relationship between adhesions and pelvic pain is controversial: the presence of pelvic adhesions is not a reliable predictor of pelvic pain; also, it has not been possible to demonstrate a relationship between the duration and severity of pain and the extent or location of adhesions[2].

In a review of the literature, analysis of uncontrolled studies by Duffy and diZerega found that adhesions can cause pelvic pain and that adhesiolysis resulted in pain relief in 60–90% of cases[16]. However, the only randomized trial of adhesiolysis failed to show any significant improvement in pain symptoms after lysis of adhesions by laparotomy, relative to a control group that did not undergo adhesiolysis. Only a subgroup of patients with severe, vascularized and dense adhesions involving the bowel had significantly more pain relief than controls[17].

Trapped ovary syndrome

Trapped ovary syndrome, or ovarian retention syndrome, is the presence of persistent pelvic pain, dyspareunia or a pelvic mass after conservation of one or both ovaries at the time of hysterectomy, and the subsequent formation of dense fibrous adhesions around the ovary. The pain is typically cyclical in nature, and should be relieved by ovarian suppression or removal.

Ovarian remnant syndrome

Ovarian remnant syndrome is defined as pelvic pain in the presence of residual ovarian tissue after oophorectomy. As the residual ovarian tissue continues to function under gonadotropin stimulation, cyclic activity and cystic changes cause pain by exerting pressure on adjacent pelvic and retroperitoneal tissues, including the posterior vagina, rectum, bladder and ureter[18]. The incidence of symptomatic ovarian remnants after oophorectomy by laparotomy is unknown[19]. An observational study by Nezhat et al.[20] showed that 13 out of 19 women who underwent laparoscopic oophorectomy had ovarian remnants. Women undergoing ovarian extirpation after piecemeal removal of the ovary during multiple previous surgeries are recognized to be at greatest risk of developing this syndrome[19]. Removing the ovarian remnant may relieve the symptoms[21].

Pelvic inflammatory disease

Pelvic inflammatory disease (PID) is a common and poorly managed disease in women of reproductive age, and presents an enormous public health and economic burden. The term chronic PID is used loosely to describe either recurrent episodes of upper genital tract infection, or residual damage caused by previous episodes of pelvic infection[11]. Residual damage caused by PID may take the form of adhesions leading to chronic pelvic pain[22]. In a review of publications on laparoscopy, chronic PID was found to account for only 5% of all diagnoses[23]. Considering the prevalence of PID and the likelihood of developing chronic pelvic pain following PID, this seems to be a low estimate of the importance of PID as the root of chronic pelvic pain. Mild PID seems to be much more common than severe or 'classic' PID, hence the importance of early recognition and treatment cannot be understated. The wide variety of clinical presentations and the lack of sensitivity and specificity of laboratory tests compound diagnostic difficulties.

Endosalpingiosis

Endosalpingiosis is defined as the presence of ectopic ciliated epithelium resembling the normal endosalpinx without endometrial stroma and involving the peritoneum or para-aortic lymph nodes. The diagnosis is rarely made preoperatively. Endosalpingiosis is often found in association with endometriosis and adenomyosis. Furthermore, the localization and gross appearance of endosalpingiosis and endometriotic lesions may appear to be the same, creating difficulty in distinguishing the difference during surgery. Visually, it appears as white to yellow, opaque or translucent, punctated and cystic lesions. A study by Heinig *et al.*[24] found that the most prevalent location of endosalpingiosis was the superficial peritoneum. Little is known about the clinical correlation of endosalpingiosis. Several studies have found that endosalpingiosis is associated with chronic pelvic pain[25,26]. deHoop *et al.* found that up to 70% of patients with endosalpingiosis suffer from chronic pelvic pain[26].

Bowel-related pain

Irritable bowel syndrome is the commonest cause of visceral pain in reproductive age women. Approximately 20% of the general population have irritable bowel syndrome. The site of pain is characteristically in the lower abdomen, particularly in the left iliac fossa, although pain may also be felt anywhere in the abdomen. The pain is characteristically cramping and variable, but at times is constant and may persist for hours or days. The variable bowel habit that characterizes irritable bowel syndrome consists of a varying frequency of defecation and, often, several early morning 'rushes' to the toilet. The stools are usually of small volume and often of variable character. Patients with irritable bowel syndrome often have associated nausea, occasional vomiting, heartburn, dyspepsia and globus syndrome. They frequently have a history of migraine and may have secondary complaints of dysmenorrhea, dyspareunia and urinary frequency[27].

Two well-known sets of diagnostic criteria for irritable bowel syndrome exist – the Manning and the Rome criteria (Table 2.2). In the Manning criteria[28], no threshold number of symptoms are recommended. The Rome criteria[29] initially specified a chronicity term of 'continuous or recurrent'; added more symptoms, with special attention to constipation-type symptoms; and required two or more of the altered defecatory patterns described in Table 2.2. Drossman *et al.* revised the Rome criteria to require one symptom to be present, as well as three or more of the altered defecatory patterns, and included a frequency requirement for pain of ≥3 months and altered defecation for ≥25% of the time[30]. Irritable bowel syndrome characteristically starts in early adult life. It is often associated with emotional and behavioral problems and appears to be related to stress in many instances[27].

Table 2.2 Diagnostic criteria for irritable bowel syndrome

Manning criteria
Abdominal pain that is relieved with a bowel movement
Pain associated with looser stools
Pain associated with more frequent stools
Sensation of incomplete evacuation
Abdominal distension

Rome criteria
Continuous or recurrent symptoms of:
Abdominal pain, relieved with defecation, or associated with a change in frequency or consistency of stool
and/or
Disturbed defecation (two or more of):
    Altered stool frequency
    Altered stool form (hard or loose/watery)
    Altered stool passage (straining or urgency, feeling of incomplete evacuation)
    Passage of mucus
usually with
    Bloating or feeling of abdominal distension

Revised Rome criteria
Continuous or recurrent symptoms for at least 3 months of:
Abdominal pain or discomfort, relieved with defecation, or associated with a change in frequency or consistency of stool
and*
An irregular (varying) pattern of defecation at least 25% of the time and three or more of:
    Altered stool frequency
    Altered stool form (hard or loose/watery)
    Altered stool passage (straining or urgency, feeling of incomplete evacuation)
    Passage of mucus
    Bloating or abdominal distension
*Comment by the committee that the decision to include the pain criterion is to be left to the discretion of investigators

Urological pain

The principal urological causes of chronic pelvic pain are interstitial cystitis and urethral syndrome. Other, more common conditions that may cause pain include chronic urinary tract infection, urethral diverticulum, urinary calculi, bladder malignancy and radiation cystitis.

Interstitial cystitis is a clinical syndrome characterized by a frequent and urgent need to urinate and/or pelvic pain in the absence of any other identifiable pathology[31]. The estimated prevalence of interstitial cystitis is between 18 per 100 000 and 510 per 100 000[31]. The etiologies of interstitial cystitis are still debated. The leading theories for pathogenesis include: changes in urothelial permeability; increased mast cell activity; neuro-immune abnormalities; neuroplasticity of the nervous system; and infectious etiology[31]. The Interstitial Cystitis Data Base Study[32] showed that almost all patients (93.6%) reported having some degree of pain. Of the patients with pain, 80.4%, 73.8% and 65.7% reported having pain in the lower abdomen, urethra and lower back, respectively. The types of pain varied, with 'pressure' and 'aching' being the most common types and 'stabbing' being the least common. Symptoms often present as episodic, and can progress to a continuous symptom of urgency or frequency with intermittent 'flares'. These flares often occur premenstrually. A more severe or end-stage bladder syndrome is sometimes seen in patients who present with disabling pain and a frequency as often as 10 minutes[31]. The gold standard in the diagnosis of interstitial cystitis is cystoscopy demonstrating characteristic appearance of submucosal oedema and petechiae. The presence of a Hunner's ulcer is pathognomonic[11]. Recently, it has been suggested that increased intravesical sensitivity to potassium chloride is sufficient for diagnosis in women with urological symptoms[33].

Chronic urethral syndrome is characterized by irritative symptoms, as well as post-void fullness and incontinence. There is evidence that urethral syndrome may be a variation of interstitial cystitis or even an early-stage interstitial cystitis[34]. The etiology is unknown, but a hypoestrogenic state, trauma or infection, particularly with chlamydia, may contribute.

Musculoskeletal pain

Research has shown that the musculoskeletal system is involved in disorders such as vulvodynia, coccygodynia, levator ani syndrome, fibromyalgia, endometriosis, vulvar vestibulitis syndrome, dyspareunia, vaginismus, pelvic floor tension myalgia, urgency–frequency syndrome, interstitial cystitis, urethral syndrome, irritable bowel syndrome and pudendal nerve entrapment/pudendal neuralgia. Whether musculoskeletal dysfunction is a primary cause of symptoms or an effect of pathology elsewhere is a crucial issue that must be addressed to achieve a successful result[35]. It is essential to examine all potential muscular and visceral sources of pain, as the symptoms of deep muscular and visceral dysfunction are often similar. The pain will most often be diffuse and accompanied by autonomic complaints. Visceral and somatic referred pain may create confusion.

Myofascial pain syndrome

Myofascial pain syndrome represents the largest group of unrecognized and undertreated acute and chronic medical problems[36]. Myofascial pain syndrome has been defined as pain that originates from myofascial trigger points in skeletal muscle. A myofascial trigger point is a hyperirritable spot, usually within a taut band of skeletal muscle or its investing fascia, that is painful upon compression and can give rise to characteristic referred pain, tenderness and autonomic phenomena. Myofascial pain syndrome may manifest as a direct result of trauma or may be an indirect result, caused by overload to compensating muscles.

Nerve-related pain

Nerve injury has been reported due to stretching, blunt trauma, compression with hypoxia, fibrosis with entrapment, or suture ligature. The incidence of postoperative neuropathies following major pelvic surgery has been reported to be 1.9%. Retractor compression injuries were the most common[37].

Common entrapment injury occurs from abdominal (iliohypogastric, ilioinguinal, genitofemoral) and pelvic (pudendal) incisions with suture ligature or fibrotic encasement. Nerve entrapments caused by suture may produce pain that can be unusually intense, localized and present immediately postoperatively. Patients may describe a pulling or a throbbing sensation for many years after the initial offending surgery. The peripheral nerve pain will often have a burning quality, and some patients may complain of shooting pain. The pain will usually become constant and more intense with time. Menstruation may also exacerbate the pain, due to perineural edema, hormone-induced increased neurotransmitters and dysmenorrhea producing dorsal horn transmission cell sensitivity. The diagnosis may be confirmed by injection of local anesthetic at the site of maximum tenderness, at the level of fascia, which should result in complete relief of pain for a variable length of time.

Other nerve-related pain includes nerve injury resulting from prolonged compression or stretching, as in the second stage of labor. Surgical injuries have also been reported with sacrospinous vaginal vault suspension, vaginal laceration repairs and various types of episiotomies. Patients have also developed pudendal neuropathy after straddle injuries, prolonged motorcycle riding and laser treatment to the vulva and perineum. The symptoms of this neuropathy range from constant burning to intense stabbing pain, and are often accompanied by pelvic floor myalgia and spasm.

Psychosocial factors

There has long been an assumption that psychological and social factors play a part in the genesis of chronic pelvic pain, but their precise role remains unclear. Researchers have attempted to find a psychopathological source for chronic pelvic pain when there is no identifiable physical cause[38]. Attempts at identifying 'psychogenic' causes for chronic pelvic pain have remained futile due to the multi-faceted nature of the problem. An immediate difficulty in the evaluation of a patient presenting with pelvic pain is gaining an understanding of how the psychosocial circumstances may have contributed to the presenting problem. Associations have been reported between chronic pelvic pain and a variety of factors, such as personality and mood disturbance, sexual and relationship difficulties, and previous adverse life experiences such as childhood events, particularly sexual abuse. The identification of such association does not prove causation. The balance between the factors will vary between patients and at different times in the course of an individual's pain.

Depression

Depression is more prevalent in women with chronic pelvic pain. Studies have shown that psychological morbidity such as depression is more likely to be a consequence rather than the cause of chronic pelvic pain[39]. Pain may contribute to or confirm a sense of helplessness or a tendency to engage in catastrophic thoughts, and may itself be exacerbated by them[40].

Sexual abuse and physical violence

A number of studies have reported an association between chronic pelvic pain and events in childhood, particularly sexual abuse. The simple cause/effect relationship between early childhood sexual abuse experiences are still inadequate to understand this condition fully. Studies have also shown that experience of physical violence tends to be higher in women with chronic pelvic pain[41].

PROTOCOL FOR INVESTIGATION

Despite all the major advances in pelvic visualization by ultrasound scan, computed tomography, magnetic resonance imaging and laparoscopy, a complete history and physical examination are the most crucial and valuable tools in the evaluation of a patient with chronic pelvic pain. The initial act of talking and listening when a patient's history is being taken establishes rapport and instils confidence in the patient, which may help in performing subsequent physical examination. It is important to remember that pelvic examination could be emotionally very stressful for a patient with chronic pelvic pain. The patient may perceive the examination as a pain aggravator.

History

The International Pelvic Pain Society has produced a useful pelvic pain assessment form for clinicians to obtain a detailed history; this form is easily obtained via their website[42]. The form not only characterizes the pain symptoms but also attempts to determine the effect of these symptoms on the patient's day-to-day functioning. However, if specific pelvic pain assessment forms are not used, then some specific questions should be asked when obtaining a history.

Firstly, the location of the pain must be determined. It is useful to have a 'pain map', which allows the patient to mark the location of pain on a picture or diagram of the body. The nature of the pain must be determined, including its severity, duration, relationship to the menstrual cycle (cyclic or non-cyclic), and aggravating and relieving factors. In clinical practice, a simple rating system of 'no pain, mild, moderate and severe pain' is often used. This system may not be very sensitive to subtle changes in pain severity and may not be useful for subsequent consultation where the patient may be reviewed by a different clinician. A more useful method involves a visual analog scale, which is often used in a research environment. In a visual analog scale, the patient places a vertical mark on a 10-cm line that most appropriately rates the pain severity, with one end being no pain and the opposite end being the most intense pain (Figure 2.1). It may be useful to ask how the patient's pain has changed over time. Establishing whether there is a temporal pattern may also be helpful. Cyclicity related to menstruation particularly suggests gynecological pain, but this is not necessarily pathognomonic of gynecological pathology. The same pattern may occur with pain of intestinal, urological or musculoskeletal origin[15]. Apart from concentrating on

Please place a vertical mark on the line to show the severity of your pain.

No pain   The most intense pain

Figure 2.1 Visual analog scale to gauge pain (line is 10 cm)

the pain itself, the history should also include bowel, urinary, general health, obstetrics, sexual and family histories (endometriosis, inflammatory bowel disease, fibromyalgia, depression, lupus, cancer). Previous surgical history may be pertinent. A history of surgery for pain is obvious, but a history of actual surgical procedure performed may provide clues other than the specific diagnosis for which the initial surgery was performed. Pregnancy and childbirth are traumatic events to the musculoskeletal system; damage to the pelvis and back may lead to chronic pelvic pain. The risk factors include lumbar lordosis, macrosomia, difficult delivery and ventouse or forceps delivery.

Screening for the impact that pelvic pain has had on the patient as an individual, her relationship and her work capacities is important. The emotional accompaniments should be measured either by history, possibly psychometric evaluation, or psychological consultation[7]. The role of psychometric instruments is to alert the clinician to problems (i.e. depression) so that the patient can be referred to a psychologist or psychiatrist. Personality profiles will not reveal a specific diagnosis but can alert the clinician to an individual's strengths and weaknesses. A social history allows the clinician to evaluate support systems and to screen for domestic violence. Victims of domestic violence have higher incidences of chronic somatic complaints, exacerbation of chronic medical conditions, chronic pain, non-compliance with medical treatment, substance abuse, anxiety, depression and suicide[43].

Physical examination

A major objective of the physical examination is to detect the exact anatomic locations of tenderness and correlate these with areas of pain. The physical examination begins as soon as the patient enters the consultation room. Usually, a patient with chronic pelvic pain will not appear visibly distressed, compared with a patient in acute pain. Close observation should be made of the patient's posture, gait, facial expression and overall general countenance. Vital signs should be taken at every clinic visit, which will provide information on general health. The particular elements of physical examination that may be included in an individual patient's examination will be dictated, in large part, by the history obtained initially.

Abdominal examination

With the patient in a supine position, the abdominal examination begins with a general inspection, looking particularly for scars or masses. The patient should be asked to point out the site of pain and then to demonstrate how much hand pressure to the area of maximal pain is needed to elicit the tenderness. Abdominal palpation should initially be superficial, noting hyperesthesia or hyperalgesia and checking for superficial abdominal reflexes. Next, careful examination of the abdominal wall in a systematic fashion for myofascial or trigger point pain is performed by single-digit palpation. When a focal tenderness is found, the patient is asked to tense the abdominal wall by raising her head and shoulders or legs off the table slightly, without the assistance of arms. If the pain elicited on single-digit palpation increases in response to the maneuver, it suggests that the pain is myofascial in origin. This test is also known by the eponym the Carnett test. Conversely, if the abdominal wall flexion reduces the pain, the source is more likely to be internal or visceral. If the pain is unchanged, this maneuver is indeterminate. Myofascial pain elicited by the Carnett test may be due to muscular strain, nerve entrapment, viral myositis, trauma, epigastric artery rupture or an abdominal wall hernia, as well as myofascial trigger points[15]. The pubic symphysis should be palpated for tenderness, suggesting symptomatic pelvic girdle relaxation, rectus muscle inflammation or injury at its fascial insertion, osteitis pubis or osteomyelitis. Other routine components of abdominal examination should not be neglected. These include examining for distension, abdominal masses and ascites, testing for shifting dullness, palpating for deep tenderness, guarding or rigidity, and auscultating for bowel sound.

Pelvic examination

The pelvic examination should begin with inspection of the external genitalia. The vulva, vestibule and urethra should be noted for redness, discharge, abscess formation, excoriation, fistulas, fissures, ulcerations, pigment changes, condylomata, atrophy or signs of trauma. Pain in this region in the absence of physical changes is often due to vulvodynia and vulvar vestibulitis, which is frequently the cause of chronic pelvic pain. A cotton-tipped swab may be used to evaluate the minor vestibular glands just external to the hymen for localized tenderness of vulvar vestibulitis. Next, a single-digit examination should be used to evaluate the vulva for trigger points. Areas of previous trauma or scars from surgeries or deliveries should be given particular attention.

Speculum examination using either a Cusco or Sims speculum will allow a full visual inspection, examination of cervical cytology and collection of bacteriological specimens. Following the speculum examination, a single-digit examination should be performed, initially to assess vaginismus, where the patient will not be able to relax the introital musculature voluntarily. Next, the pelvic floor musculatures are evaluated. Many patients have painful spasms of the pelvic floor musculature, including the levator ani, obturator, pubococcygeus and deep transverse perineal muscles; sometimes specific trigger points can be identified. The finger is then rotated anteriorly to palpate, initially with a single digit and then bimanually, the anterior vaginal wall, urethra and base of the bladder to elicit any areas of tenderness, induration, discharge or thickening, which might suggest chronic urethritis, chronic urethral syndrome, urethral diverticulum, vaginal wall cyst, trigonitis or interstitial cystitis. The cervix, paracervical areas and vaginal fornices should also be palpated for tenderness to elicit problems such as cervical trauma, pelvic infection, endometriosis, urethral pain and trigger points. Pelvic floor pain may be a primary problem or it may be secondary to other diseases, such as interstitial cystitis or endometriosis. The uterus is assessed bimanually to evaluate for tenderness, which could be due to adenomyosis or pelvic infection. A fixed and immobile uterus may suggest endometriosis or adhesion. Rectal or rectovaginal examination should be performed last. Marked discomfort on rectal examination may indicate chronic constipation or irritable bowel syndrome. In patients with pudendal nerve injury, the perineum should also be evaluated for areas of hypoesthesia or paraesthesia.

Diagnostic tests

The choice of diagnostic test used to evaluate chronic pelvic pain will be dictated by the history and physical examination. Table 2.3 lists some of the tests that may be used to evaluate the more common causes of chronic pelvic pain. Diagnostic and therapeutic endoscopies, such as laparoscopy, hysteroscopy, colonoscopy or cystoscopy, are useful only when visceral causes of pain are suspected[2].

The laparoscope has traditionally been considered the gold standard for the diagnosis of chronic pelvic pain. A survey of published series suggests that over 40% of diagnostic laparoscopies by gynecologists are performed for chronic pelvic

Table 2.3 Tests that may be used to evaluate common causes of chronic pelvic pain

Adhesions	Ultrasonography, hysterosalpingography, magnetic resonance imaging, laparoscopy
Adenomyosis, fibroids	Ultrasonography, hysterosalpingography, magnetic resonance imaging, hysteroscopy, laparoscopy
Chronic urethral syndrome	Urodynamic test
Diarrhea	Stool specimens for ova and parasites, stool culture, stool for *Clostridium difficile* toxin, barium enema, colonoscopy, computed tomography
Diverticular disease	Barium enema
Dyspareunia	Urethral and cervical cultures for gonorrhea, ultrasonography, laparoscopy
Endometriosis	Blood for CA 125, ultrasonography, computed tomography, magnetic resonance imaging, laparoscopy
Endosalpingiosis	Laparoscopy
Hernias	Abdominal wall sonography, computed tomography
Interstitial cystitis	Cystoscopy, potassium chloride challenge tests, urine bacteriological culture, urine cytology, urodynamic test, bladder biopsy
Ovarian remnant syndrome	Blood hormone profile (FSH, estradiol), ultrasonography, computed tomography, laparoscopy
Pelvic congestion syndrome	Pelvic venography, ultrasonography
Pathology of cervix	Colposcopy
Porphyria	Urine porphobilinogen
Trapped ovary syndrome	Ultrasonography, computed tomography, laparoscopy
Urethral diverticulum	Vaginal ultrasound, cystourethrography, magnetic resonance imaging
Urinary calculi	Abdominal X-ray
Vulvodynia	Colposcopy

FSH, follicle-stimulating hormone

pain[44]. The incidence of abnormal findings at laparoscopy is 35–83%[5]. Endometriosis and adhesions account for at least 85% of all laparoscopic findings[15]. However, it is important to remember that it does not automatically follow that identified pathology is causally related to pain. It is also true that a negative laparoscopy is not synonymous with no pathology or no physical basis for pain. Laparoscopy might be most useful when there is a high index of suspicion for endometriosis, with severe dysmenorrhea, dyspareunia and pouch of Douglas nodularity.

A different diagnostic laparoscopic approach, termed 'conscious laparoscopic pain mapping', has been advocated by several authors to improve the diagnostic capability. This approach is performed under local anesthesia, with or without conscious sedation, with the goal of identifying sources of pain in women with chronic pelvic pain. The technique involves gentle probing of tissues, lesions and organs with a blunt probe. Diagnosis is based on the severity of pain elicited and on the replication of the pain that is the patient's presenting symptom. This method appears attractive but currently there are too few data confirming its diagnostic accuracy.

Cystoscopy is advocated if chronic pelvic pain is suspected to be originating from the bladder. Diagnosis of interstitial cystitis is made with the combination of clinical history and cystoscopy. As mentioned earlier, the appearance of submucosal edema and petechiae is associated with interstitial cystitis. Other clinical criteria include irritative voiding symptoms, such as frequency, urgency and nocturia. However, microscopic hematuria and infection should be ruled out first prior to cystoscopy, due to the non-invasiveness of the tests required, which are urinary microscopy and urine culture. Discovery of hematuria is a definite indication for cystoscopy to rule out malignancy.

Radiological tests commonly used to evaluate chronic pelvic pain include ultrasonography and saline infusion sonography, computed tomography, magnetic resonance imaging and, less commonly, hysterosalpingography. Each has inherent advantages and disadvantages. Transvaginal ultrasound and, less often, transabdominal ultrasound, are frequently the initial imaging techniques used to evaluate women with chronic pelvic pain. Ultrasonography is extremely sensitive for detecting fluid collection, but areas of fat, air, bone or other various non-fluid densities in the scanning plane may inhibit transmission of a clear image[45]. Sonohysterography is a procedure in which sterile saline is infused into the uterine cavity transcervically followed by a transvaginal ultrasound examination. Sonohysterography allows evaluation of the endometrial cavity, where it can delineate polyps, endometrial cancer and submucosal fibroids[45]. The role of computed tomography is limited in the evaluation of women with chronic pelvic pain, due to the associated ionizing radiation and limited contrast resolution. However, computed tomography can provide global assessment of the abdomen and pelvis, which can provide organ-specific information. Magnetic resonance imaging is especially useful for characterizing and determining the origin of an adnexal mass, such as endometrioma, pedunculated subserous fibroid and dermoid, and diagnosing uterine abnormalities. Specifically, magnetic resonance imaging is the best technique to diagnose adenomyosis and for distinguishing it from fibroids. Hysterosalpingography permits evaluation of uterine–tubal patency as well as any subtle distortions of the uterine cavity.

CONCLUSIONS

Chronic pelvic pain is a serious problem. It is an enigmatic syndrome that is the complex interplay of biological and psychosocial phenomena. Diagnosis can be difficult, and both the clinician and the patient may have difficulty accepting the diagnosis. Initial accurate assessment is both essential and crucial to obtain a correct diagnosis. This initial correct diagnosis will hopefully lead to proper management so that patients with chronic pelvic pain do not enter a lengthy trail of seeing one specialist after another and avoid unnecessary re-investigations.

REFERENCES

1. International Association for the Study of Pain. Definition of Pain. In Merskey H, Bogduk N, eds. IASP Pain Terminology. Seattle: IASP Press, 1994.

2. Howard FM. The role of laparoscopy in the chronic pelvic pain patient. Clin Obstet Gynecol 2003; 46: 749–66.

3. Zondervan K, Yudkin P, Vessey M, et al. Prevalence and incidence in primary care of chronic pelvic pain in women: evidence from a national general practice database. Br J Obstet Gynaecol 1999; 106: 1149–55.

4. Zondervan K, Barlow DH. Epidemiology of chronic pelvic pain. Bailliere's Best Pract Res Clin Obstet Gynaecol 2000; 14: 403–14.

5. Gunter J. Chronic pelvic pain: An integrated approach to diagnosis and treatment. Obstet Gynecol Surv 2003; 58: 615–23.

6. Gambone JC, Mittman BS, Munro MG, et al. The Chronic Pelvic Pain/ Endometriosis Working Group. Consensus statement for the management of chronic pelvic pain and endometriosis: proceedings of an expert-panel consensus process. Fertil Steril 2002; 78: 961–72.

7. Steege JF. Office assessment of chronic pelvic pain. Clin Obstet Gynecol 1997; 40: 554–63.

8. Fukaya T, Hoshiai H, Yajima A. Is pelvic endometriosis always associated with chronic pain? A retrospective study of 618 cases diagnosed by laparoscopy. Am J Obstet Gynecol 1993; 169: 719–22.

9. Moen M, Stokstad T. A long term follow up study of women with asymptomatic endometriosis diagnosed incidentally at sterilization. Fertil Steril 2002; 78: 961–72.

10. Nisolle M, Donnez J. Peritoneal endometriosis, ovarian endometriosis, and adeno-myotic nodules of the rectovaginal septum are three different entities. Fertil Steril 1997; 68: 585–96.

11. Moore J, Kennedy S. Causes of chronic pelvic pain. Bailliere's Best Pract Res Clin Obstet Gynaecol 2000; 14: 389–402.

12. Stones RW. Pelvic vascular congestion – half a century later. Clin Obstet Gynecol 2003; 46: 831–6.

13. Beard R, Reginald P, Wadsworth J. Clinical features of women with chronic lower abdominal pain and pelvic congestion. Br J Obstet Gynaecol 1988; 95: 153–61.

14. Beard RW, Stones RW. Chronic pelvic pain: the gynaecologist's perspective. In O'Brien PMS, ed. The Yearbook of Obstetrics and Gynaecology. London: RCOG Press, 1999: 76–86.

15. Howard FM. Chronic pelvic pain. Obstet Gynecol 2003; 101: 594–611.

16. Duffy D, diZerega G. Adhesion controversies: pelvic pain as a cause of adhesions, crystalloids in preventing them. J Reprod Med 1996; 41: 19–26.

17. Peters A, Trimbos-Kemper G, Admiraal C, Trimbos J. A randomised clinical trial on the benefit of adhesiolysis in patients with intraperitoneal adhesions and chronic pelvic pain. Br J Obstet Gynaecol 1992; 99: 59–62.

18.   Symmonds R, Pettit P. Ovarian remnant syndrome. Obstet Gynecol 1979; 54: 174–7.

19.   Webb M. Ovarian remnant syndrome. Aust NZ Obstet Gynaecol 1989; 29: 433–5.

20.   Nezhat CH, Seidman DS, Nezhat FR, et al. Ovarian remnant syndrome after laparoscopic oophorectomy. Fertil Steril 2000; 74: 1024–8.

21.   Siddall-Allum J. The ovarian remnant syndrome. J Royal Soc Med 1994; 87: 375–6.

22.   Munday PE. Clinical aspects of pelvic inflammatory disease. Hum Reprod 1997; 12 (11 Suppl): 121–6.

23.   Howard FM. The role of laparoscopy as a diagnostic tool in chronic pelvic pain. Bailliere's Best Pract Res Clin Obstet Gynaecol 2000; 14: 467–94.

24.   Heinig J, Gottschalk I, Cirkel U, Diallo R. Endosalpingiosis – an underestimated cause of chronic pelvic pain or an accidental finding? A retrospective study of 16 cases. Eur J Obstet Gynecol Reprod Biol 2002; 103: 75–8.

25.   Keltz M, Kliman H, Arici A, Olive D. Endosalpingiosis found at laparoscopy for chronic pelvic pain. Fertil Steril 1995; 64: 482–5.

26.   deHoop T, Mira J, Thomas M. Endosalpingiosis and chronic pelvic pain. J Reprod Med 1997; 42: 613–16.

27.   Swarbrick E. Chronic pelvic pain: the physician's perspective. In O'Brien PMS, ed. The Yearbook of Obstetrics and Gynaecology. London: RCOG Press, 1999: 66–75.

28.   Manning AP, Thompson WG, Heaton KW, Morris AF. Towards positive diagnosis of the irritable bowel. Br Med J 1978; 2: 653–4.

29.   Thompson W, Dotevall G, Drossman D, et al. Irritable bowel syndrome: guidelines for diagnosis. Gastroenterol Int 1989; 2: 92–5.

30.   Drossman D, Thompson W, Talley N, et al. Identification of subgroups of functional gastrointestinal disorders. Gastroenterol Int 1990; 3: 159–72.

31.   Butrick CW. Interstitial cystitis and chronic pelvic pain: new insights in neuropathology, diagnosis, and treatment. Clin Obstet Gynecol 2003; 46: 811–23.

32.   Simon LJ, Landis R, Erickson DR, Nyberg LM, The ICDB Study Group. The Interstitial Cystitis Data Base Study: Concepts and preliminary baseline descriptive statistics. Urology 1997; 49 (Supplement 5A): 64–75.

33.   Parsons C, Bullen M, Kahn B, et al. Gynecologic presentation of interstitial cystitis as detected by intravesical potassium sensitivity. Obstet Gynecol 2001; 98: 127–32.

34.   Parsons C. Prostatitis, interstitial cystitis, chronic pelvic pain, and urethral syndrome share a common pathophysiology: lower urinary dysfunctional epithelium and potassium recycling. Urology 2003; 62: 976–82.

35.   Prendergast SA, Weiss JM. Screening for musculoskeletal causes of pelvic pain. Clin Obstet Gynecol 2003; 46: 773–82.

36.   Rosen N. The myofascial syndromes. Phys Med Rehabil Clin N Am 1993; 4: 41–63.

37.   Perry CP. Peripheral neuropathies and pelvic pain: diagnosis and management. Clin Obstet Gynecol 2003; 46: 789–96.

38.   Savidge C, Slade P. Psychological aspects of chronic pelvic pain. J Psychosom Res 1997; 42: 433–44.

39.   McGowan L. Chronic pelvic pain: a meta-analytical review. Psychol Health 1998; 13: 937–51.

40.   Stones RW, Selfe SA, Fransman S, Horn SA. Psychological and economic impact of chronic pelvic pain. Bailliere's Best Pract Res Clin Obstet Gynaecol 2000; 14: 415–31.

41.   Walling MK, Reiter RC, O'Hara MW, et al. Abuse history and chronic pain in women: l. Prevalences of sexual abuse and physical abuse. Obstet Gynecol 1994; 84: 193–9.

42.   The International Pelvic Pain Society Research Committee. Pelvic pain assessment form. The International Pelvic Pain Society. http:// www.pelvicpain.org.

43.   Eisenstat S, Bancroft L. Domestic violence. N Engl J Med 1999; 341: 886–92.

44.   Howard FM. The role of laparoscopy in chronic pelvic pain: promise and pitfalls. Obstet Gynecol Surv 1993; 48: 357–87.

45.   Cody RF, Ascher SM. Diagnostic value of radiological tests in chronic pelvic pain. Bailliere's Best Pract Res Clin Obstet Gynaecol 2000; 14: 433–66.

3

Role of conscious laparoscopic pain mapping in the management of women with chronic pelvic pain

Ying Cheong, Raya Al-Talib, R William Stones

INTRODUCTION

Conscious laparoscopic pain mapping (CLPM) is a diagnostic laparoscopy performed under local anesthesia in women with chronic pelvic pain; the objective is to localize the sources of tenderness with the aid of the patient when a mechanical stimulus is applied to areas in the pelvis and the pelvic organs. Some studies have shown that this procedure helps in the diagnosis of unusual or subtle pathology that would not normally be diagnosed under general anesthesia[1,2], although the latter claim remains controversial[3]. However, there has been a continued interest in CLPM in the management of women with chronic pelvic pain, albeit not as a first-line investigation.

CONSCIOUS LAPAROSCOPIC PAIN MAPPING – THE SOUTHAMPTON EXPERIENCE

Princess Anne Hospital (PAH) in Southampton is a tertiary referral center for the management of chronic pelvic pain. In a recent observational study[4] of women who had CLPM over the last 4 years, 51% ($n = 20$) were referred from general practitioners, 36% ($n = 14$) were inter-hospital referrals and 13% ($n = 5$) were intra-hospital referrals. The average duration of pelvic pain in this group of women at the time of referral to PAH was 38 months (SD = 43), which is not surprising given that a large study conducted in Oxfordshire ($n = 483$) has shown that the vast majority of women who have troublesome pelvic pain symptoms delay seeking medical help[5].

Of the women who were referred and who had CLPM, 80% ($n = 30$) had already undergone at least one laparoscopy, 31% ($n = 12$) had undergone at least one laparotomy (Table 3.1), 13% ($n = 5$) had undergone operative laparoscopy and 5% ($n = 2$) had had vaginal surgery. In a proportion of this group of women who had undergone surgery, pathology had been found ($n = 9$; 23%) and had already been treated. In total, 95% ($n = 37$) of women had received various medical treatments before pain mapping; these treatments were: progestogens ($n = 12$; 31%); combined oral contraceptives ($n = 12$; 31%); gonadotropin-releasing hormone agonists ($n = 5$; 13%); and others such as danazol and gabapentin ($n = 8$; 21%) (Figure 3.1).

In practice, patients who were selected for CLPM were a specific subgroup in whom, following a clinical history and examination, the assessment was that CLPM would be able to identify a problem that could be resolved by further surgery and/or that the presence of generalized, non-localized tenderness might enable the patient to reorient her goals toward pain management, rather than a search for specific focal pathology. No black-and-white rules exist in the selection of these women for CLPM; rather, the process is seen as very much dependent on the consultation and the goals and expectations of the individual patient. In particular, given the unpleasantness of the procedure, it is only to be considered when positively desired by the patient after full counseling.

PATIENT SELECTION AND THE PROCEDURE

The procedure can be rather uncomfortable and women selected to undergo CLPM should be able to tolerate Trendelenburg's position and ideally, should not be obese. Steege has suggested using the 'belly grab' test to assess a patient's suitability for CLPM[6]. The few contraindications to CLPM include severe cardiopulmonary conditions such as severe chronic obstructive airway disease, pulmonary hypertension and heart failure. Patients who have had previous anesthetic complications are also not ideal candidates. We have performed all our CLPM procedures in theater with anesthesia back-up. Normally, when CLPM has proved technically difficult, we have abandoned the procedure rather than convert to general anesthesia.

Prior to CLPM, the woman should be counseled about the nature of the procedure. She should know that it will be performed in theater under local anesthesia to the skin, and that two surgical incisions (one subumbilical and one suprapubic) will be made during surgery. Sedation is given via an intravenous injection (Table 3.2) and an anesthetist is present. The procedure can be stopped any time the patient wishes so she is the one in control. The risks of a laparoscopy – including visceral injury, laparotomy under general anesthesia and failure of the procedure due to technical difficulties of entry, insufflation or an obscured view

Table 3.1 Number and frequency of pre-conscious laparoscopic pain mapping laparoscopies and laparotomies in women referred to Princess Anne Hospital for the management of chronic pelvic pain

	Frequency	
	n	(%)
Number of laparoscopies		
before referral (n)		
0	9	23
1	17	44
2	9	23
3	3	8
4	1	3
Total	39	100
Number of laparotomies		
before referral (n)		
1	10	26
2	2	5
Total	12	31

caused by adhesions – should be explained clearly before embarking on the procedure, with the aid of an information sheet. The patient needs to fast for 6 hours prior to the operation, and consent should be obtained for additional necessary procedures, such as general anesthesia and laparotomy, in case of an emergency.

The patient is required to empty her bladder immediately prior to the operation, avoiding the need for catheterization. The surgeon should talk the patient through the injection of the local anesthetics and the insertion of the Veress needle; the additional insertion of the primary trocar can be avoided by using a port expander. The secondary trocar should be inserted under direct vision. Initial experience was gained with the 2-mm mini-laparoscope but this proved fragile and gave suboptimal views, and was therefore abandoned. Some procedures have been undertaken using the 10-mm operating laparoscope, with a port inserted through the operating channel, obviating the need for a suprapubic puncture. The authors' current preferred instrumentation is a 5-mm laparoscope inserted via the port expander with the use of a suprapubic puncture for probing. Manipulation of the uterus is achieved by placement of Hulka tenaculum forceps, after infiltration of the cervix with Citanest. Warming up of all instruments prior

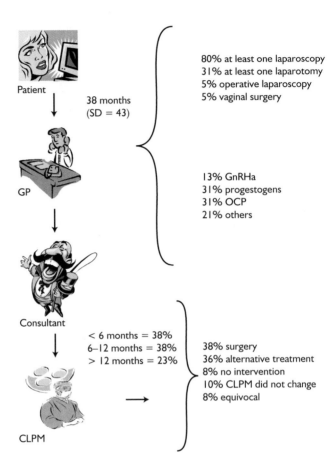

Patient

38 months
(SD = 43)

80% at least one laparoscopy
31% at least one laparotomy
5% operative laparoscopy
5% vaginal surgery

GP

13% GnRHa
31% progestogens
31% OCP
21% others

Consultant

< 6 months = 38%
6–12 months = 38%
> 12 months = 23%

38% surgery
36% alternative treatment
8% no intervention
10% CLPM did not change
8% equivocal

CLPM

Figure 3.1 Conscious laparoscopic pain mapping – the patient's journey. GP, general practitioner; CLPM, conscious laparoscopic pain mapping; GnRH, gonadotropin-releasing hormone agonist; OCP, oral contraceptive pill

to their use is critical to patient comfort. The gas insufflation pressure limit should be reduced to 10 mmHg.

Bupivicaine 0.25% should be infiltrated into the puncture sites in the anesthetic room on arrival of the patient. The anesthetist then inserts an intravenous cannula and a small initial dose of midazolam is given. After the patient has been transferred to the operating theater, she is positioned and connected to a pulse oximeter and blood pressure cuff. Oxygen is then given via a transparent facemask. Further increments of midazolam and fentanyl can be given during the procedure as required. Our unit's protocol is shown in Figure 3.2.

Table 3.2 Types and dosage of anxiolytics and narcotics available for use in conscious laparoscopic pain mapping

	Suggested dosage
Anxiolytic	
Diazepam	0.05–0.15 mg/kg at 2.5 mg every 5 min
Midazolam	0.02–0.07 mg/kg at 1.0 mg every 5 min
Narcotic	
Fentanyl	1–3 mg/kg at 25–50 mg every 5 min
Alfentanil	250–500 mg/kg at 5–10 mg every 5 min
Morphine	0.1–0.15 mg/kg at 1–2 mg every 5 min

The pelvis should initially be inspected for pathology, bearing in mind that pathology such as endometriosis can be subtle. Occult pathology, such as femoral, inguinal and sciatic hernias, also need to be considered[7]. Such hernias are repairable laparoscopically. The entire pelvis should be examined systematically for tenderness on mechanical stimulation, and a pain score should be elicited from the patient. Local injection of tender points on the anterior abdominal wall and specific areas such as the vault can be performed during CLPM. The patient can then be assessed as to whether the local anesthetic injection has alleviated the pain. This procedure of local injection to abdominal wall tenderness can then be repeated in an outpatient setting if the patient found it helpful intraoperatively. However, it is important to document the exact point of injection for reference at a later date, and to bear in mind during the procedure that there is a normal pattern of tenderness of the pelvic organs, including lateralization of sensation[8].

LIMITATIONS OF CONSCIOUS LAPAROSCOPIC PAIN MAPPING

Although CLPM has the advantage of the patient being conscious, thereby allowing her to alert the clinician to the site of tenderness, the assumption could be made that pain stimulus in chronic pelvic pain must be mechanical. This, in fact, has not been fully supported by the literature. The pathophysiology of pain in chronic pelvic pain is often not mechanical. There has been little research on the actual effect of laparoscopy and gaseous insufflation on pain perception. Furthermore, even when pathology such as endometriosis has been diagnosed,

Indications
Chronic pelvic pain.
No contraindications to standard day-case laparoscopy, especially excessive weight or midline scar.

Preoperative preparation
At preoperative assessment
Information sheet, if not already given; answer queries; record weight.
Give bowel prep: two Picolax sachets for day before surgery, taken with plenty of water.
Advise fasting from midnight (for morning list).

In waiting area
Review by anesthetist; consent form signed.
Note LMP.
Pass urine immediately before transfer to theater to avoid need for catheterization.

In anesthetic room
Small iv cannula sited.
Midazolam iv 2 mg over 30 s.
Fentanyl 50 μg iv (1 ml of 50 μg/ml solution).
0.25% bupivicaine rectus block at two lateral sites (10 ml each) plus subumbilical infiltration (10 ml)
with orange needle.
Further 10 ml 0.25% bupivicaine at suprapubic puncture site if this portal is to be used. Mark site with
pain.

In theater
Lloyd–Davies position; blanket over abdomen at this stage. Use warm instruments. Arms at sides or
extended.

Clean, drape and expose cervix with Sims' speculum. Citanest (prilocine plus octapressin) intracervical
injection at four cardinal points with dental syringe. Place Hulka tenaculum forceps on cervix.

Expose abdomen, clean, drape. Use warm instruments. Subumbilical puncture with Veress needle.
Insufflate approximately 1.5 l CO_2 or nitrous oxide with pressure regulator set at maximum 7 mmHg.

Place subumbilical trocar and cannula. Attach camera and commence video recording. Second
puncture if required, or probe via laparoscope operating channel.

Record pain levels at different sites in the pelvis on 0–10 verbal rating scale. Offer patient the
opportunity to view the monitor and direct the examination if she wishes.

Discontinue insufflation; take care to remove the gas from the peritoneal cavity. Suture skin puncture
sites if required. Consider Voltarol depending on concomitant medication and degree of discomfort
after instruments removed.

Indications for conversion to GA
Suspected bowel or vascular injury; suspected pelvic or abdominal pathology not fully evaluated under
LA; patient request (consider abandoning procedure rather than converting to GA).

Throughout the procedure:
Pulse oximetry and blood pressure monitor.
Further increments of 0.5–1 μg midazolam to a total maximum of 5 mg
(= 83 μg/kg for a 60 kg woman).
Further increments of 50 μg Fentanyl up to total maximum 200 μg.

GA, general anesthesia; LA, local anesthesia; LMP, last menstrual period

Figure 3.2 Southampton's surgical protocol for pain mapping

the pain correlation with mechanical stimulus to the affected areas has been inconsistent[1].

However, the findings of CLPM could help guide the clinician on the subsequent steps in the management of chronic pelvic pain. A study on all the women who underwent pain mapping over the last 4 years in Southampton showed that tenderness occurred in the following areas, in decreasing order of frequency: ovaries and/or uterus (38%; $n = 15$); generalized hyperalgesia, therefore suggesting neuropathic pain (21%; $n = 8$); adhesions and sterilization clip (13%; $n = 5$); abdominal wall (8%; $n = 3$); occult inguinal hernia (8%; $n = 3$); vaginal vault (5%; $n = 2$); and others (5%; $n = 2$)[4].

POST-CONSCIOUS LAPAROSCOPIC PAIN MAPPING (CLPM) MANAGEMENT OF CHRONIC PELVIC PAIN

As a result of these findings, we were able to triage women who had CLPM for further surgery (41%; $n = 16$), further hormonal treatment (28%; $n = 11$) or

Table 3.3 Outcomes of conscious laparoscopic pain mapping (CLPM): case-note-based rating of 'success' and 'failure'

	%	n
Success (n = 32)		
Procedure identified a problem amenable to surgery and patient was better after recommended surgery	38	15
Procedure indicated that surgery was going to be unhelpful; patient had alternative therapy and improved	36	14
Patient was better informed and reassured	8	3
Failure (n = 4)		
Adhesions were removed but no improvement	3	1
Failed attempt of embolization of pelvic veins and patient lost to follow-up	3	1
CLPM suggested abdominal wall tenderness; local injection of area did not work	5	2
Equivocal (n = 3)		
Patient became pregnant, therefore treatment stopped	3	1
Recommended surgery but patient lost to follow-up	5	2

further pain management via the multidisciplinary pain team (26%; $n = 10$); 5% ($n = 2$) were discharged back to their general practitioner. Defining 'success' as the outcome of benefit to the patient (Table 3.3), we concluded, on the basis of the case-note review, that 82% of the procedures were successful.

CONCLUSIONS

Although CLPM should not be embarked upon as a first-line investigation in women with chronic pelvic pain, it has a specific role in the management ladder. Appropriate history and examination, in combination with an individual-focused approach to each woman in terms of meeting her expectations and goals in the short, intermediate and long term, are vital. Before CLPM, the woman should be well informed. Under these conditions, the procedure could be helpful in moving the patient's treatment forward.

REFERENCES

1. Almeida OD, Val-Gallas JM. Conscious pain mapping. J Am Assoc Gynecol Laparosc 1997; 4: 587–90.

2. Demco LA . Effect on negative laparoscopy rate in chronic pelvic pain patients using patient assisted laparoscopy. J Soc Laparoendosc Surg 1997; 1: 319–21.

3. Palter SF, Olive DL. Office microlaparoscopy under local anesthesia for chronic pelvic pain. J Am Assoc Gynecol Laparosc 1996; 3: 359–64.

4. Cheong YC, Stones RW. Role of conscious laparoscopic pain mapping – mapping out the patient's journey. Abstract. British Society for Gynaecological Endoscopy. Dublin; 2004.

5. Zondervan KT, Yudkin PL, Vessey MP, et al. Patterns of diagnosis and referral in women consulting for chronic pelvic pain in UK primary care. Br J Obstet Gynaecol 2001; 106: 1156–61.

6. Steege JF. Microlaparoscopy. In Steege JF, Metzger DA, Levy BS, eds. Chronic Pelvic Pain. Philadelphia: WB Saunders Company, 1998.

7. Howard F. The role of laparoscopy in the chronic pelvic pain patient. In Sharp H, ed. Clinical Obstetrics and Gynecology. Vol. 46. Philadelphia: Lippincott Williams and Wilkins, 2003: 749–66.

8. Koninckx P, Renaer M. Pain sensitivity and pain radiation from the internal female genital organs. Hum Reprod 1997; 12: 1785–8.

4 | Adhesions and chronic pelvic pain

Ying Cheong, Tin-Chiu Li

INTRODUCTION

Chronic pelvic pain is a substantial healthcare problem. In the primary care setting, the annual prevalence (38/1000) was found to be comparable to conditions such as asthma (37/1000) and back pain (41/1000)[1]. In the hospital setting, chronic pelvic pain was found in 39% of women undergoing sterilization and subfertility investigations[2]; this high rate may be skewed by population bias but, nevertheless, chronic pelvic pain is an important healthcare issue in the UK.

One of the important causes of chronic pelvic pain is pelvic adhesion. Adhesions are scar tissue resulting from previous trauma/inflammation. Although there are many recognized causes of adhesions – including bacterial peritonitis, radiotherapy, chemical peritonitis, foreign body reaction, long-term continuous ambulatory peritoneal dialysis, endometriosis and pelvic inflammatory disease – the majority of adhesions occur following surgery.

To further our understanding of the possible relationship between adhesions and pain, it is important initially to understand what adhesions are.

WHAT ARE ADHESIONS?

Adhesions are 'internal scars' that form after trauma through complex processes, involving the interaction between injured tissues and the peritoneum. Adhesion tissue is a mixture of macrophages, eosinophils, red blood cells, tissue debris, mast cells, fibroblasts and nerve tissue.

The etiology of adhesions can be divided into three main catogories: congenital; infectious; and postsurgical. Congenital adhesions rarely give rise to adhesion-related morbidity. Conditions such as pelvic inflammatory disease, appendicitis, diverticulitis and inflammatory bowel disease are examples of infective conditions capable of inducing adhesions. The most common cause of peritoneal adhesions is prior surgery, although autopsy studies reveal about 30% prevalence of some adhesions in women who have never had surgery[3]. Postoperative adhesion development has been reported to occur in 55–100% of patients after surgery[4–11]. In order of increasing frequency, the anatomical sites for postoperative adhesion formation at second-look laparoscopy have been found to be: the ovary (71%); pelvic sidewall (76%); and anterior parietal peritoneum beneath the abdominal incision (94%)[12–14].

ADHESION FORMATION

Adhesion formation involves trauma to the peritoneum, which is covered by mesothelial cells. Mesothelial cells are loosely attached to the basement membrane and can be readily detached by the slightest trauma[15]. In the event of trauma, the area of injury mounts an acute inflammatory response, which involves inflammatory cells such as neutrophils and macrophages, whose functions are mediated by various cellular mediators[16–19].

After trauma/injury to the peritoneum, there is increased vascular permeability in vessels supplying the damaged area, followed by an exudation of inflammatory cells, ultimately leading to the formation of a fibrin matrix. The fibrin matrix is gradually organized and replaced by tissue containing fibroblasts, macrophages and giant cells. This fibrin matrix connects two injured peritoneal surfaces forming fibrin bands. These fibrin bands can be broken down by fibrinolysis into smaller molecules[3] – fibrin degradation products (FDP[4]). Under conditions of aberrant peritoneal healing, ischemia results in a reduction in fibrinolytic activity and thus the persistence of the fibrin bands. The organization of the fibrin bands over time results in persistence of the adhesions (Figure 4.1).

Newly formed adhesions at 48 hours post-laparoscopic adhesiolysis are filmy, relatively soft and avascular in nature. They are easily lysed by gentle traction to the surrounding organs to which they are attached, such as the bowels or ovaries. They are present in areas where the peritoneum has been denuded or traumatized. The areas where adhesions are re-formed are bloodless, with the occasional old blood clot but no active bleeding/ooze[18].

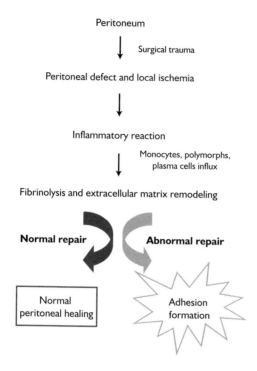

Figure 4.1 A summary of normal tissue repair and adhesion formation following surgical trauma. After trauma to the peritoneum, an inflammatory reaction at the site of injury is evoked and the influx of the cellular components involved in inflammation occurs. Depending on the processes of inflammation, fibrinolysis and extracellular matrix remodeling, normal or abnormal healing can result, the latter leading to adhesion formation

DO ADHESIONS CAUSE PAIN?

A meta-analysis of over 3000 women with chronic pelvic pain and over 2000 controls showed that adhesions are present in 36% of women with chronic pelvic pain compared to 15% of controls[20]. The important question, however, is whether the association between adhesions and pelvic pain is casual or causal. Unfortunately, the question of whether adhesions cause pain does not currently have a satisfactory answer. Some declare that it is an 'unsubstantiated myth' that adhesions cause pain,[21] while others think that 'adhesions can cause pelvic pain and adhesiolysis relieves it in 60–90% of the cases'[22]. It therefore appears that some adhesions are associated with pain and some not.

Peters *et al.* proposed that adhesions that are dense and vascular are more likely to result in pelvic pain[23]. Others believed that the peritoneum, when under traction and tension, produces pain as a result of activation of pain receptors in the adhesion tissue and the viscera. To date, the best evidence that adhesions can cause pain comes from Kresch *et al.*[24]. In this study, the investigators compared 100 women with pelvic pain for a minimum period of 6 months with a control group of 50 asymptomatic women who were undergoing laparoscopic sterilization. In the 100 women with chronic pelvic pain, 48% had adhesions involving their uterus, ovaries and bowel, and 32% had endometriosis, while in the control group, 14% had adhesions and 15% had endometriosis. The investigators also observed that the adhesions in the control group were loose and did not restrict bowel mobility, whilst adhesions in the group of women with chronic pelvic pain were more restrictive of the mobility of the viscera. In this study, the one important patient inclusion criterion was that the pain needed to be in a consistent location, regardless of its character. This criterion was not always used in many other studies. Furthermore, some organs, such as the ovaries, are richly innervated, and during processes such as ovulation produce the long-recognized phenomenon of mittelschmerz (ovulation pain). Similarly, when the ovary has been trapped or stretched by adhesions, pain can result.

More interestingly, it has been shown that adhesion tissue contains nerve fibers. Kligman *et al.* obtained adhesion tissue from 17 patients, 10 with chronic pain and seven without, and examined the tissue by immunohistochemistry for nerve tissues; 10 of the 17 specimens contained nerve fibers[25]. The nerve fibers were evenly distributed between patients with and without pain. Tulandi *et al.* performed a similar but larger study on 50 patients and found no difference in the amount and quantity of nerve fibers in adhesions from women with and without pelvic pain[26]. However, Tulandi *et al.* remarked on the limitations of the study: based on a 77% proportion of nerve fibers in women without pelvic pain, to detect a 10% difference in the proportion of nerve fibers in the two groups of women with a 5% level of significance and a power of 80%, a total of 502 women (251 women in each group) is needed. Therefore, the two studies to date that have examined nerve fibers and adhesion tissue did not have enough power to answer the question.

Nevertheless, the findings that adhesion tissues contain nerves may help explain why only some adhesions cause pain. Adhesions that are stretched during movement of the viscera can result in stimulation of the pain fibers, thus initiating the release of chemical mediators and pain response.

TREATMENT OF ADHESIONS

A number of non-randomized studies have shown that division of adhesions at surgery is useful in the treatment of chronic pelvic pain[27–30]. In terms of retrospective studies, a meta-analysis showed that of over 600 patients with chronic pelvic pain, 76% would obtain relief from adhesiolysis (Table 4.1). According to data from prospective studies, 51% of women would obtain relief of their pelvic pain from adhesiolysis[23,28,31] (Table 4.2).

CRITICAL ANALYSIS OF STUDIES ON ADHESIOLYSIS

Central and local causes

Before commencing an analysis of the effect of adhesiolysis, one should understand that chronic pelvic pain has central and local causes. Although pain can be initiated by a peripheral stimulus, eventually there exists a central modulation so much so that even after the initial stimulus has disappeared, the perception of pain still exists, such as in the case of the phantom limb. The exact timing of the onset of the stimulus of pain is difficult to obtain and standardise in studies. Many studies do not include psychological morbidity, which again is strongly linked to patients' perception of pain[32].

Placebo effect: the grateful patient syndrome

Surgery is almost inevitably associated with some degree of placebo effect. A good doctor–patient relationship can induce a powerful placebo effect[33]. The most recent study on adhesiolysis and chronic abdominal pain[31] reviewed a 27% placebo effect in both the study and the control groups. This effect is often long-lasting, and studies examining the effect of adhesiolysis on pain should have a follow-up period of at least 1 year, which is often not the case.

Types of adhesions

As discussed before, adhesion type may predict whether adhesions cause pain or not. Therefore, studies looking into the effect of adhesiolysis should classify the adhesions in study patients in terms of their site, severity and extent. It should

Table 4.1 Retrospective studies of adhesiolysis in women with pelvic pain

Reference	No. of patients	Surgery	Cured or improved	Same or worse
Goldstein et al., 1980	18	Microsurgery (9) Laparoscopy (9)	16 (89%)	2(11%)
Kleinhaus, 1984	2	Laparoscopy	2 (100%)	—
Chan et al., 1985	43	Microsurgery	28 (65%)	14 (33%)
Mecke et al., 1988	39	Laparoscopy	23 (59%)	16 (41%)
Daniel, 1989	42	Laparoscopy	28 (67%)	14 (33%)
MacDonald & Sutton, 1992	118	Laparoscopy	91 (77%)	27 (17%)
Fayaz et al., 1994	156	Laparoscopy	(97%)	(3%)
Sarevalos et al., 1995	123	Microsurgery (72) Laparoscopy (51)	82 (66%)	18 (34%)
Mueller et al., 1995	45	Laparoscopy	30 (66%)	6 (13%)
Nezhat et al., 2000	48	Laparoscopy	32 (67%)	16 (33%)
Schietroma et al., 2001	45	Laparoscopy	34 (83%)	7 (17%)
Total	679		76%	24%

also be noted whether adhesions are attached tightly or loosely to visceral or nerve-rich structures such as the ovaries.

Other pathology

Pathology such as endometriosis or ongoing pelvic infection can be a source of pelvic pain. Therefore, studies examining the effect of adhesiolysis should exclude such conditions by careful history-taking, examination and, if laparoscopy is performed, careful inspection for early endometriosis, which may only be evident to the experienced eye (see below).

Adhesion recurrence

Up to 90% of adhesions can re-form after they are lysed, and this re-formation can occur very early[18]. Many studies, however, failed to perform second-look

Table 4.2 Prospective studies of adhesiolysis in women with pelvic pain

Reference	No. of patients	Surgery	Cured or improved	Length of follow-up (months)
Steege and Stout[28] (1991)	30	Laparotomy	40–70%	6–12
Peters et al.,[23] (1992)	48	Laparotomy	38–42%	9–12
Swank et al.,[31] (2003)	100	Laparoscopy	42–57%	12

laparoscopy to evaluate the effectiveness of the surgery. These studies also did not use adjuvants to prevent adhesion formation. If adhesions re-form, then, surely, patients' pain can recur.

WHY THERE IS A NEED FOR A RANDOMIZED CONTROLLED TRIAL ON GYNECOLOGICAL PATIENTS WITH CHRONIC PELVIC PAIN

There have been many retrospective studies on the effects of adhesiolysis, but without randomization, observational studies are subject to many drawbacks. Of the three prospective studies, only one randomized controlled trial has evaluated the benefits of adhesiolysis for chronic abdominal and pelvic pain[31]. This trial was performed in patients with chronic abdominal pain recruited from various hospitals in The Netherlands. The investigators performed adhesiolysis in 100 patients (87% female, 13% male), and post-surgical evaluation was carried out for up to 12 months. The authors found no difference in pain scores denoted by the VAS (Visual Analog Scale), SF-36 (36-item short-form health survey) and the MQS (Medical Qualification Scale) between the treatment group and the control group. They also found a large placebo effect of 27% after surgery.

Although this trial was robustly conducted, there was no information on the presence or absence of gynecological pathology such as endometriosis or pelvic inflammatory disease. The exclusion criteria were mainly concerned with abdominal pathology, including abnormal abdominal but not pelvic computed tomography (CT) or ultrasound scans. This is an important point, because even among experienced gynecologists, endometriotic changes can be very subtle and difficult to diagnose, and endometriosis is a known cause of pelvic pain. Moreover, endometriosis involving the ovarian fossae should be carefully inspected, because restriction of the mobility of the ovaries may also be a contributing factor in chronic pelvic pain, analogous to that caused by residual ovary syndrome whereby the ovary is encased by adhesions (usually postoperative) and functional physiological ovarian cyst formation results in pain. Other pelvic disease not detectable by radiological scans, such as pelvic congestion and pelvic inflammatory disease, were also not mentioned in the study of Swank *et al.*[31].

Differentiation between pelvic and abdominal pain

Gynecologists diagnose and treat pelvic pain rather than abdominal pain. The location of pelvic pain is usually within the anatomical pelvis, below the umbilicus, and occasionally around the lower back. The main symptoms of pelvic pain also include dysmenorrhea and/or dyspareunia. The investigation and management pathways concerning women with pelvic pain, dysmenorrhea and dyspareunia, for obvious reasons, are very different from those in patients with abdominal pain with gastroenterological symptomatology. The problem of overlap between gynecological and gastroenterological pathology and symptoms needs continuing evaluation, and hence the importance of obtaining a good history (with a review of all systems) and examination cannot be overemphasized. The latter, however, is time-consuming, and hence such patients should be seen in a specialist clinic in a multidisciplinary setting[34], where time can be spent especially on the first consultation, and further evaluation of the chronic pelvic pain performed by a psychotherapist, specialist nurse and physiotherapist where appropriate (Figure 4.2). Specialists in different fields should work together so that patients with such overlapping symptoms can obtain maximum input from the gynecologist and gastroenterologist as well as the surgeon.

Site, extent and severity of adhesions

Although we know that an ischemic injury resulting in an inflammatory response can cause adhesion formation, the modulation process of adhesion formation/reformation resulting in different natures of adhesions is still poorly understood. Similarly, although it is known that adhesions contain nerves, little is known about the quality or quantity of nerve tissue in different types of adhesions[26]. In essence, the pathophysiology of adhesion formation, and whether adhesion formation is a progressive disease, are still poorly understood. Thus, adhesions should be systematically typed according to the site, because this will allow

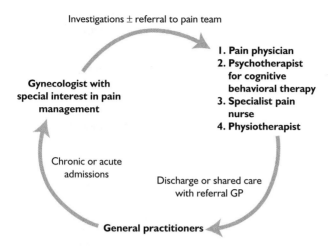

Investigations ± referral to pain team

Gynecologist with
special interest in pain
management

1. **Pain physician**
2. **Psychotherapist
   for cognitive
   behavioral therapy**
3. **Specialist pain
   nurse**
4. **Physiotherapist**

Chronic or acute
admissions

Discharge or shared care
with referral GP

General practitioners

Figure 4.2 Flow chart of referral and management of women with chronic pelvic pain within the multidisciplinary team setting

further definition of whether adhesions at certain sites cause pain more than others. For example, if adhesiolysis were to be performed around the ovaries to allow their mobility to be resumed, would pain relief be more substantial compared with lysing similarly extensive adhesions on the uterus or anterior abdominal wall? Demco assessed the relationship between adhesions and pain during concious microlaparoscopic pain mapping[35]. This author found that filmy adhesions between mobile structures such as the ovaries cause more pain than dense, fixed adhesions. This, however, contradicts the results of Peters *et al.* which showed that dense, severe adhesions are more likely to responsed to adhesiolysis treatment than filmy, mild ones[23]. Therefore, the relationship between adhesions and pain is more complex than just in terms of site, severity and extent.

Psychological factors and assessment

Psychological assessment is important in the management of chronic pain conditions. Treating the physical pain alone can leave emotional and evaluative issues unresolved, and possibly exacerbate them through reinforcement. Swank *et al.*[31] excluded women with a history of psychological problems and patients on medications that stimulate the central nervous system, mainly because such patients are more prone to having psychogenic chronic pain. Gradually emerging knowledge indicates that a whole host of somatic, psychological and socioenvironmental factors may act and interact in its causation, together forming a multidimensional 'biopsychosocial' model of disease etiology. Thus, psychological assessment of patients undergoing investigations and treatment for chronic pelvic pain is important. In a research setting, mere exclusion of this group of patients is not practical, because adhesions may have been the cause rather than the result of their chronic pelvic pain. Prior knowledge of their psychological status allows the planning of further multidisciplinary management. Steege and Stout[28] performed adhesiolysis in women with chronic pain syndrome and women without. Women with chronic pain syndrome responded significantly less well after adhesiolysis than women without chronic pain syndrome, and the authors suggested that the presence of 'psychosocial compromise warrants preoperative evaluation and concomitant treatment'. If the psychosocial well-being of a patient is important in their response to surgery, then surely such patients should undergo preoperative evaluation before surgery and the results should be corrected for this confounding factor.

PREVENTION OF ADHESION FORMATION/RE-FORMATION

Currently, there is no ideal method of preventing adhesion formation/re-formation. In terms of surgical technique, gentle tissue handling, meticulous hemostasis, copious irrigation, prevention of infection, avoidance of powdered gloves (which can evoke a foreign body response in the peritoneum) and prevention of extensive thermal injury have all been described as means of adhesion prevention.

Adjuvants to prevent postsurgical adhesion have also been evaluated. They include agents that prevent inflammation, such as steroidal and non-steroidal anti-inflammatory medications, agents that degrade fibrin, such as recombinant tissue plasminogen activator, and barrier methods involving the application of an absorbable material/solution/gel intraperitoneally to prevent the peritoneal surfaces from adhering together[36]. Two early commercially available synthetic barriers for adhesion prevention, namely oxidized regenerated cellulose (Interceed, Johnson and Johnson, Ethicon Inc., Somerville, NJ) and polytetrafluoroethylene (WL Gore & Associates Inc., Flagstaff, AZ), have both been shown to be safe and efficacious in reducing the incidence of postoperative adhesions[37]. Interceed (TC 7) Absorbable Adhesion Barrier (Ethicon Inc.) is absorbable and can be cut to the size required to cover a surgical field without suturing. It needs to be placed on the raw tissue area after adequate hemostasis has been achieved. The other commercially available barrier is Gore-Tex (WL Gore & Associates Inc.), which is non-absorbable and needs to be sutured in place, and has the disadvantage that it needs to be removed during a subsequent surgical procedure. Though meta-analyses have shown that these adhesion prevention barriers are capable of reducing adhesions after surgery, they do not completely eliminate the formation and re-formation of adhesions in all patients.

Seprafilm (Hal-F, Bioresorbable Membrane, Genzyme Corporation, Cambridge, MA) is an adhesion barrier derived from sodium hyaluronate and carboxymethylcellulose. It is absorbed from the peritoneal cavity within 7 days and excreted from the body within 28 days. Randomized controlled trials to date have shown that Seprafilm reduces the incidence, extent and severity of adhesions, compared with controls[38–40]. Sepracoat (HAL-C, Genzyme Corporation) is a liquid that coats the organs that it comes into contact with. A randomized controlled trial on 277 patients undergoing gynecological surgery via laparotomy has shown that it effectively reduces adhesions, although more studies are required to confirm this finding.

Intergel (Ethicon Inc.) is a 0.5% ferric hyaluronate gel that acts as an anti-adhesion barrier. It is derived from hyaluronic acid, a natural component of the fluid that lubricates the human joints, and has been shown to reduce adhesions by 59–69%[41,42]. However, it has recently been withdrawn from the market pending investigations into the circumstances surrounding some adverse events, including postoperative pain and inflammatory reactions. There were also two deaths where the product was used after accidental puncture of the bowel.

Icodextrin solution (Adept; Shire Pharmaceuticals, Basingstoke, UK) has recently been evaluated for its effectiveness in adhesion prevention. For many years, icodextrin has been used in patients with peritoneal dialysis. Up to a liter of the solution is instilled into the peritoneal cavity and hydrofloatation prevents raw organ surfaces from opposing after surgery, reducing adhesion formation/re-formation. In a pilot randomized controlled trial of 62 patients, Adept was found to reduce adhesion formation, compared with Ringer's Lactate[43]. More recent adhesion barriers include a sprayable hydrogel, SprayGel (Confluent Surgical Inc., Waltham, MA). SprayGel consists of two polyethylene glycol (PEG)-based liquids (clear and blue procurers) that mix together within seconds to form a biocompatible absorbable hydrogel; hence, when sprayed onto tissue, the gel adheres to the tissue to form a flexible barrier which is later hydrolyzed and re-absorbed by the body after 5–7 days and is cleared by the kidneys. This gel can be applied to open as well as endoscopic procedures and initial studies have shown promising results[44,45].

CONCLUSIONS

Intra-abdominal adhesions are a diagnosis that needs to be borne in mind whilst women are investigated and treated for chronic pelvic pain. Some patients will benefit from adhesiolysis. However, adhesion re-formation remains a difficult problem to resolve. It is important that we have in the future robust trials to evaluate the role of adhesiolysis in gynecological patients, and such trials should consider psychological evaluation and multidisciplinary management packages. Although there are many different commercially available products for adhesion prevention, there is currently no one product that can significantly reduce adhesion formation/re-formation. Research is ongoing into other means of reducing adhesions, such as alteration of cellular mediators[16] and the fibrinolytic pathway[46]. Until we learn to cover the footprints of surgery, adhesion prevention strategies will still rely on good surgical techniques and meticulous hemostatic control.

REFERENCES

1. Peters A, Bakkum E, Hellebrekers B. Clinical significance of adhesions in patients with chronic pelvic pain. In Maclean A, Stones R, Thornton S, eds. Pain in Obstetrics and Gynaecology. London: RCOG press, 2001: 214–23.

2. Mahmood T, Templeton A, Thomson L, Fraser C. Menstrual symptoms in women with pelvic endometriosis. Br J Obstet Gynaecol 1991; 98: 558–63.

3. Weibel M, Majno G. Peritoneal adhesions and their relation to abdominal surgery. A post mortem study. Am J Surg 1973; 126: 345–53.

4. Raj S, Hulka J. Second-look laparoscopy in infertility surgery: therapeutics and prognostic value. Fertil Steril 1982; 49: 26.

5. Diamond M, Feste J, Mclaughlin D. Pelvic adhesions at early second-look laparoscopy following carbon dioxide laser surgery. Infertility 1984; 7: 39–44.

6.   Diamond M, Daniel J, Johns D. Postoperative adhesion development following operative laparoscopy: evaluation at early second-look procedures. Fertil Steril 1991; 55: 700–4.

7.   DeCherney A, Mezer H. The nature of posttuboplasty pelvic adhesions as determined by early and late laparoscopy. Fertil Steril 1984; 41: 643–6.

8.   Daniell J, Pittaway D. Short-interval second-look laparoscopy after infertility surgery: a preliminary report. J Reprod Med 1983; 28: 281–3.

9.   Surrey M, Friedman S. Second-look laparoscopy after constructive pelvic surgery for infertility. J Reprod Med 1982; 27: 658–60.

10.   Trimbos-Kemper T, Trimbos J, vanHall E. Adhesion formation after tubal surgery: results of the eighth-day laparoscopy in 188 patients. Fertil Steril 1985; 43: 395–400.

11.   Pitttaway D, Daniell J, Maxson W. Ovarian surgery in an infertility patient as an indication for a short-interval second-look laparoscopy: a preliminary study. Fertil Steril 1985; 44: 611–14.

12.   Azziz R. Pelvic sidewall adhesion reformation: microsurgery alone or with Interceed absorbable adhesion barrier. Surg Gynecol Obstet 1993; 177: 135–9.

13.   Becker J, Dayton M, Fazio V, et al. Prevention of post-operative abdominal adhesions by sodium hyaluronate-based bioresorbable membrane: a prospective, randomised, double-blind multicentre study. J Am Coll Surg 1996; 183: 297–306.

14.   Franklin R, Diamond M, Malinak L, et al. Reduction of ovarian adhesions by the use of Interceed. Obstet Gynecol 1995; 86: 335–40.

15.   Raftery A. Regeneration of parietal and visceral peritoneum in the immature animal: a light and electronmicroscopical study. Br J Surg 1973; 60: 969–75.

16.   Cheong YC, Laird S, Shelton JB, et al. Peritoneal healing and adhesion formation/reformation. Hum Reprod Update 2001; 7: 556–66.

17.   Cheong YC, Laird SM, Shelton JB, et al. The concentrations of IL-1, IL-6 and TNF-alpha in the peritoneal fluid of women with pelvic adhesions. Hum Reprod 2001; 17: 69–75.

18.   Cheong YC, Laird SM, Shelton JB, et al. The correlation of adhesions and peritoneal fluid cytokine concentrations: a pilot study. Hum Reprod 2002; 17: 1039–45.

19. Cheong Y, Shelton J, Laird S, et al. Peritoneal fluid concentrations of matrix metalloproteinase-9, tissue inhibitor of metalloproteinase-1 and transforming growth factor-beta in women with pelvic adhesions. Fertil Steril 2003; 79: 1168–75.

20. Saravelos H, Li T, Cooke I. Adhesions and chronic pelvic pain. Contemp Rev Obstet Gynaecol 1995; 7: 172–7

21. Alexander-Williams J. Do adhesions cause pain? Br Med J (Clin Res Ed) 1987; 294: 659–60.

22. Duffy D, diZerega G. Adhesion controversies: pelvic pain as a cause of adhesions, crystalloids in preventing them. J Reprod Med 1996; 41: 19–26.

23. Peters A, Trimbos-Kemper G, Admiraal C, et al. A randomised clinical trial on the benefit of adhesiolysis in patients with intraperitoneal adhesions and chronic pelvic pain. Br J Obstet Gynaecol 1992; 99: 59–62.

24. Kresch A, Seifer D, Sachs L, et al. Laparoscopy in 100 women with chronic pelvic pain. Obstet Gynecol 1984; 64: 672–4.

25. Kligman I, Drachenberg C, Papadimitriou J, Katz E. Immunohistochemical demonstration of nerve fibres in pelvic adhesions. Obstet Gynecol 1993; 82: 566–8.

26. Tulandi T, Chen M, Al-Took S, Watkin K. A study of nerve fibers and histopathology of postsurgical, postinfectious, and endometriosis-related adhesions. Obstet Gynecol 1998; 92: 766–8.

27. Mueller M, Tshudi J, Herrmann U, Klaiber C. An evaluation of laparoscopic adhesiolysis in patients with chronic abdominal pain. Surg Endosc 1995; 9: 802–4.

28. Steege J, Stout A. Resolution of chronic pelvic pain after laproscopic lysis of adhesions. Am J Obstet Gynecol 1991; 165: 278–81.

29. Sutton C, MacDonald R. Laser laparosocpic adhesiolysis. J Gynecol Surg 1990; 6: 155–9.

30. Saravelos H, Li T, Cooke I. An analysis of the outcome of microsurgical and laparoscopic adhesiolysis for chronic pelvic pain. Hum Reprod 1995; 10: 2895–901.

31. Swank D, Swank-Bordewijk S, Hop W, et al. Laparoscopic adhesiolysis in patients with chronic abdominal pain: a blinded randomised controlled multi-centre trial. Lancet 2003; 361: 1247–51.

32. Hansen G, Streltzer J. The psychology of pain. Emerg Med Clin North Am 2005; 23: 339–48.

33. Bruxelle J. Placebo effect in the treatment of pain. Rev Pract 1994; 15: 1919–23.

34. Cheong Y, Stones W. Optimising health services for women with adhesion-related chronic pelvic pain. Adhesions News Views 2005; (7): 18–20.

35. Demco L. Pain mapping of adhesions. J Am Assoc Gynecol Laparosc 2004; 11: 181–3.

36. diZerega GS. Use of adhesion prevention barriers in pelvic reconstructive and gynaecological surgery. In diZerega GS, ed. Peritoneal Surgery. New York: Springer-Verlag, 1999: 379–99.

37. Farquhar C, Vandekerckhove P, Watson A, et al. Barrier agents for preventing adhesions after surgery for subfertility. The Cochrane Library (The Cochrane Collaboration). Cochrane Database Syst Rev 2000; (4): CD000475.

38. Vrijland W, Tseng L, Eijkman H, et al. Fewer intraperitoneal adhesions with use of hyaluronic acid-carboxymethylcellulose membrane: a randomized clinical trial. Ann Surg 2002; 235: 193–9.

39. Beck D. The role of Seprafilm bioresorbable membrane in adhesion prevention. Eur J Suppl 1997; 577: 49–55.

40. Diamond M. Reduction of adhesions after uterine myomectomy by suprafilm membrane (HAL-F): a blinded, prospective, randomised, multicenter clinical study. Fertil Steril 1996; 66: 904–10.

41. Johns D, Keyport G, Hoehler F, diZerega G, Intergel Adhesion Prevention Study Group. Reduction of postsurgical adhesions with Intergel adhesion prevention solution: a multicenter study of safety and efficacy after conservative gynecologic surgery. Fertil Steril 2001; 76: 595–604.

42. Lundorff P, van Geldorp H, Tronstad S, et al. Reduction of post-surgical adhesions with ferric hyaluronate gel: a European study. Hum Reprod 2001; 16: 1982–8.

43. diZerega G, Verco S, Young P, et al. A randomized, controlled pilot study of the safety and efficacy of 4% icodextrin solution in the reduction of adhesions following laparoscopic gynaecological surgery. Hum Reprod 2002; 17: 1031–8.

44. Johns D, Ferland R, Dunn R. Initial feasibility study of a sprayable hydrogel adhesion barrier system in patients undergoing laparoscopic ovarian surgery. J Am Assoc Gynecol Laparosc 2003; 10: 334–8.

45. Mettler L, Auderbert A, Lehmann-Willenbrock E, et al. Prospective clinical trial of SprayGel as a barrier to adhesion formation: an interim analysis. J Am Assoc Gynecol Laparosc 2003; 10: 339–44.

46. Holmdahl L. The plasmin system, a marker of the propensity to develop adhesions. In diZerega G, ed. Peritoneal Surgery. New York: Springer-Verlag, 1999: 117–31.

5 | The management of rectovaginal endometriosis

Tin-Chiu Li, Hany Lashen, Ian Adam, Yat May Wong

INTRODUCTION

Rectovaginal endometriosis is a severe form of endometriosis with a high morbidity. It is a rare condition and its presentation may be missed by the unwary. The treatment of this condition can be challenging. Medical therapy of this form of endometriosis is of limited value. Complete surgical excision of the endometriotic tissue is the cornerstone of successful treatment. From time to time it also involves bowel resection. In this chapter we highlight the presentation, treatment and outcome of the various methods of managing this condition.

WHAT IS RECTOVAGINAL ENDOMETRIOSIS?

Endometriosis of the rectovaginal septum is a form of deeply infiltrating endometriosis involving a specific location: the rectovaginal septum (Figure 5.1). Approximately 5% of all endometriosis cases involve the large bowel and, of these cases, 76% involve the rectum or rectosigmoid area[1]. Rectovaginal endometriosis is relatively uncommon, comprising approximately 3% of all cases of endometriosis[2]. It represents an advanced and often an active stage of endometriosis.

Donnez et al.[3] have recently proposed that this disease be renamed as rectovaginal adenomyosis because histologically, the rectovaginal nodule resembles an adenomyoma.

Adenomyoma is a circumscribed nodular aggregate of smooth muscle, endometrial glands and stroma. It is characterized by the presence of abundant muscular tissue invaded by glandular epithelium and covered with scanty stroma. The invasion of the muscle by a very active glandular epithelium proves that stroma is not necessary for the invasion in adenomyosis. They suggested that this specific disease originates from the Müllerian rests present in the rectovaginal septum. Adenomyosis often does not respond to physiological levels of

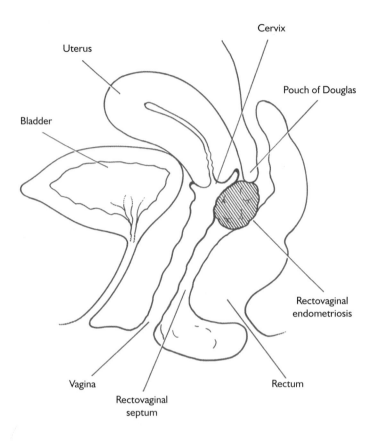

Figure 5.1 Anatomy of the rectovaginal septum and rectovaginal endometriosis, which is situated at the top or upper third of the septum. It may, from time to time, be missed by a casual laparoscopic inspection of the pelvis. Combined per rectal and per vaginal examination is necessary to ascertain the diagnosis and assess the extent of the disease

progesterone and secretory changes are often absent or incomplete during the second half of the menstrual cycle.

The presence of deep endometriosis is strongly correlated with pelvic pain. Like cystic ovarian endometriosis, it is associated with an increased level of serum CA 125 and placental protein 14, with decreased plasma natural killer cell activity[4], unlike superficial endometriosis which is associated with a mainly increased level of CA 125 in the peritoneal fluid. While cystic ovarian endometriosis is strongly associated with pelvic adhesions, deeply infiltrating rectovaginal endometriosis is not generally associated with such adhesions.

In the revised American Fertility Society classification, ovarian cystic endometriosis is normally classified as Stage 3 and 4, while deeply infiltrating endometriosis often comes under Stage 1 and 2 because of lack of adhesions[5]. Hence, the conventional scoring system does not reflect the severity of the disease in this situation. Rectovaginal endometriosis has the tendency of spreading laterally up and around the uterine artery and can also cause fibrosis around the ureter. Therefore, a thorough preoperative assessment of the extent of the disease is essential to ensure a successful outcome in the management of this condition.

MALIGNANT TRANSFORMATION

Rectovaginal endometriosis may undergo malignant transformation, and the rectovaginal septum has the highest tendency for malignant transformation in extragonadal endometriosis, with a three-fold increase in risk[6]. Whilst the overall risk of malignancy is still low, a biopsy of the lesion should be obtained to exclude malignant change if conservative/expectant treatment is to be considered or if it is deemed necessary to defer surgical treatment. Moreover, rectovaginal endometriosis may sometimes mimic carcinoma of the rectum, which is another important reason why biopsy of the lesion is desirable if conservative treatment is adopted.

PRESENTATION

Symptoms

Rectovaginal endometriosis characteristically presents as severe deep dyspareunia, referred to the rectum or lower sacral regions, severe pelvic pain and dysmenorrhea. It may penetrate through the vaginal wall producing a polyp-like deep blue hemorrhagic lesion causing irregular vaginal bleeding. Rectovaginal endometriosis may also present as cyclical rectal bleeding, discomfort on defecation (indicating bowel involvement) and, rarely, colonic or rectal obstruction. It may mimic rectal carcinoma in its presentation.

Signs

Speculum examination may reveal the presence of blue-domed cysts in the posterior fornix. On bimanual digital examination, painful nodules in the rectovaginal septum or pouch of Douglas may be detected. On rectal examination, tenderness may be elicited at the rectovaginal septum and the rectum may be fixed. A combined rectovaginal examination performed simultaneously using the index and middle fingers, especially at the time of menstruation, is the most sensitive method of detecting rectovaginal endometriosis.

INVESTIGATIONS

Preoperative investigations

Sigmoidoscopy

Rigid rather than flexible sigmoidoscopy is preferred as it may serve as an extension of the examiner's finger in 'palpating' firm masses on the rectal wall. This area will also be tender when it is manipulated with the sigmoidoscope. As rectal carcinoma is a differential diagnosis in most cases of suspected rectovaginal endometriosis, a preoperative sigmoidoscopy is mandatory in the management of this condition.

This procedure is best carried out at the time of menstruation, as the finding is most reliable at this stage of the menstrual cycle. While endometriosis rarely invades through the intestinal mucosa, an intact mucosa will effectively rule out rectal carcinoma. Rigid sigmoidoscopy may show mucosal distortion secondary to submucosal infiltration. The mucosa may also be flattened or puckered with loss of mobility from its underlying muscularis. Extrinsic fixation and angulation of the rectosigmoid colon is another common finding during sigmoidoscopy. Endoscopic biopsy rarely confirms the diagnosis of endometriosis[7].

Barium enema

Donnez *et al.* have recommended air contrast barium enema to evaluate the extent of infiltration of the anterior rectal wall[3]. Similarly, March and Israel advocated barium enema examination in addition to sigmoidoscopy prior to embarking on surgery for rectovaginal endometriosis[8]. It is not uncommon to find additional segments of the large bowel involved with severe disease leading to a scarred and constricted lumen.

Intravenous urogram

An intravenous urogram is advisable preoperatively, as it may identify any distortion of the urinary tract involved with endometriosis. This will help in the intraoperative management of the urinary tract system and allows liaison with the urologist if necessary.

Imaging

Abdominal and ultrasound scans have not been shown to be sensitive enough to diagnose this condition[4]. However, with the advance in magnetic resonance imaging (MRI) technology in recent years, this method of imaging has increasingly been used to diagnose rectovaginal septum endometriosis and to assess urinary tract and bowel involvement. Although MRI may detect lesions more than 1 cm in size, smaller lesions may be missed. Another method of detecting rectovaginal septum endometriosis is by transrectal ultrasonography[9], but further evaluation of this particular method is required.

CA 125

Plasma CA 125 measurement has been used to diagnose deeply infiltrating endometriosis. The blood sample is best obtained at the onset of menstruation. The use of CA 125 measurement has been advocated by Koninckx and Martin[4] who, using 35 U/ml as the cut-off value, reported a sensitivity of 36% and specificity of 87%. Overall, the value of CA 125 in the diagnosis and evaluation of endometriosis in general, and rectovaginal endometriosis in particular, is rather limited.

Laparoscopy

Laparoscopy may reveal the presence of pelvic endometriosis and bowel involvement of the disease. Rectal retraction at the cervix may sometimes be the only feature visible on laparoscopy. However, the diagnosis may easily be missed, especially if the lesion is small. Cul-de-sac obliteration may not be apparent during laparoscopy.

Biopsy

The final confirmation of the diagnosis still rests with histological confirmation of a biopsy specimen. Leiman *et al.* proposed that fine-needle aspiration cytology of the palpable nodule and a Tru-Cut biopsy of the mass is a simple method of making the diagnosis[2].

TREATMENT

The treatment of rectovaginal endometriosis depends on a number of factors, including the patient's age, parity, menopausal status, extent of disease and her childbearing desire.

Medical therapy

The value of medical treatment in the management of rectovaginal endometriosis is uncertain. Hormonal treatment, e.g. down-regulation of the pituitary–ovarian axis by a gonadotropin-releasing hormone analog or danazol, may suppress active endometriotic lesions may not help pain arising from scarring and fibrosis of the lesions. However, in young women with endometriosis involving only the rectovaginal septum but not the rest of the pelvis, and who wish to preserve their fertility, conservative treatment may be an option and should be discussed along with the pros and cons of surgical intervention. If the symptoms in these women are not particularly distressing, there may be an argument for a trial of medical treatment (hormonal treatment and analgesia). In contrast, in women who have already completed their family and who have severe symptoms, surgical treatment is advisable.

Pre- and postoperative medical therapy

To date, there are no clinical data to show whether pre- or postoperative medical treatments influence the outcome of surgical treatment of rectovaginal endometriosis. The prospective trial by Koninckx and Martin[4] in the management of deeply infiltrating disease with a gonadotropin analog 3 months prior to surgery, compared with a controlled arm, was terminated early when it was found that the treated group had easier surgical excision with less bleeding. However, this study did not specifically include patients with rectovaginal endometriosis. In our own small retrospective series ($n = 14$), in those patients who had been given preoperative medical therapy, there was no indication to suggest that their operation was easier to perform (unpublished data). It is not uncommon to find that these patients, who eventually had surgical management, have had prolonged medical therapy prior to their operation. Donnez *et al.* postulated that as the disease behaves more like adenomyosis than endometriosis, the response to steroids is unpredictable and often unsuccessful[3]. Similarly, there are no data to suggest that postoperative adjuvant medical treatment improves outcome.

Surgery

Surgery is the ultimate treatment for rectovaginal endometriosis. The basic principle for a successful surgical procedure is to resect all the visible and detectable endometriosis/adenomyosis lesions whenever technically possible, while preserving fertility whenever feasible and desired by the patient. Every step should be taken during surgery to minimize tissue injury and prevent adhesion formation. Hence, the principles of microsurgery should be closely adhered to, including: gentle tissue handling; constant irrigation and suction to avoid tissue desiccation; and meticulous hemostasis[10,11].

Preoperative bowel preparation and antibiotics

Preoperative bowel preparation is essential to reduce the morbidity and complications that are associated with bowel surgery. It has been a routine practice in our unit to prescribe Picolax (Nordic, Langley, Berkshire, UK) – one sachet twice a day – the day before the operation. Prophylactic antibiotics usually comprise cefuroxime and metronidazole.

Laparotomy or laparoscopy

Traditionally, surgical management of rectovaginal endometriosis involves a laparotomy.

Recently, laparoscopic management of rectovaginal endometriosis has been proposed[1,12]. The advantages of laparoscopic surgery are a shorter recovery period, a less painful recovery period, no major abdominal wall incisions, reduction in postoperative hospital stay and improved cosmetic results. However, laparoscopic surgery in rectovaginal endometriosis takes a longer operating time than a laparotomy, requires advanced skills and is currently limited to only a few centers with the expertise in minimal access surgery. With a longer operating time, complications – e.g. compartment syndrome (a condition in which prolonged compression on the calf leads to ischemia and muscle infarction) of the legs – can ensue when the patient has been in a prolonged lithotomy position.

There are a number of reasons why some gynecologists still prefer to carry out the excision of rectovaginal endometriosis via laparotomy. Firstly, the surgery is difficult and often bloody, and to carry out the surgery laparoscopically requires very advanced laparoscopic skills. Secondly, careful palpation of the tissue is necessary for accurate definition of the extent of the disease and hence the excision margins. It also helps to determine what type of bowel surgery (if any) is required. Thirdly, if there is lateral extension to the bowel or ureters, the colorectal surgeons and urologists may not be comfortable carrying out complex surgery via the laparoscope.

Combined laparoscopic and vaginal colpotomy

It is possible that rectovaginal endometriosis may be removed via the vaginal approach[13]. However, careful laparoscopic inspection to exclude involvement of the sigmoid colon is a prerequisite. In general, the removal of rectovaginal endometriosis via the vaginal route is advisable only in small lesions involving the lower part of the septum.

Hysterectomy and oophorectomy

Hysterectomy and bilateral oophorectomy may not cure rectovaginal endometriosis, although it is often performed in women with endometriosis who have failed to respond to more conservative measures. The most important surgical principle in the management of rectovaginal endometriosis is the complete excision of any fibrotic as well as active endometriotic lesions[1,12,14–16]. Hysterectomy and bilateral oophorectomy may help to prevent recurrence of the disease, provided that all lesions have been completely excised[17]. A common problem encountered in the surgery of rectovaginal endometriosis is fibrosis involving the pouch of Douglas, making total hysterectomy a very difficult procedure, resulting in a subtotal hysterectomy being performed instead. This is not advisable as it only removes the uterus, which is normal and not involved in endometriosis, leaving the fibrotic lesions with active endometriosis behind.

Resection of vaginal lesions

From time to time, part of the vaginal wall that is involved in rectovaginal endometriosis may need to be excised to ensure complete resection of the disease.

Should colorectal surgeons be involved in the surgical treatment of rectovaginal endometriosis?

In our unit, the standard practice is to carry out the operation jointly with a colorectal surgeon. We believe that the care and outcome are much better with joint management. As the disease commonly affects the muscularis layer of the bowel, a gynecologist who operates on the bowel on an infrequent basis may not be proficient in this type of surgery. Medico-legal considerations may also be important if bowel complication does occur following surgery. Our approach is also favored by Bailey et al.[7]. However, gynecologists who consider themselves proficient with bowel surgery may continue to operate independently without regular assistance from colorectal surgeons[1].

Bowel surgery

Bowel resection is not always a necessity during the surgical management of rectovaginal endometriosis. If the endometriosis is small and superficial, excision of the nodule from the rectovaginal septum is all that is required. Endometriotic lesions that are not firmly adherent to the bowel mucosa may simply be dissected and excised without the need for any anastomosis or repair. Endometriotic nodules that are firmly attached to or have penetrated the bowel mucosa require local bowel resection or more extensive resection. Anterior resection is necessary in situations where the upper part of the rectum is involved. Primary anastomosis may be carried out if the bowel has been adequately prepared preoperatively, if deemed appropriate. Otherwise, a temporary colostomy should be performed to protect the resected bowel margin's integrity. Patients who are undergoing surgical management for their rectovaginal endometriosis ought to be seen and counseled by the colorectal surgeon about the possibility of a colostomy/ileostomy.

Avoiding ureteric injury during surgical management

The appreciation of the involvement of the ureters with endometriosis is essential for preventing injury to these structures during operation. Rectovaginal endometriosis may spread laterally and cause fibrosis of tissues around the ureters. Hence, an intravenous urogram preoperatively is useful to identify any involvement of the ureters. During the dissection of rectovaginal endometriosis, it is important to stay medial to the uterosacral ligaments at all times, as the ureter normally lies lateral to these ligaments[1]. The entire course of the ureter must be identified if there is any doubt about its anatomical position.

Secondly, diathermy or vaporization of endometriotic lesions overlying the ureters ought to be avoided. Dissection and excision of the lesion is to be preferred[1]. The technique of hydroprotection may be employed prior to excision; the overlying peritoneum can be injected with fluid to lift it off the ureter from the surrounding tissues[18–20].

Finally, if there is any doubt about the position of the ureters, a stent may be inserted into each ureter, allowing easy identification of the structures during operation.

How can a rectal perforation be excluded or confirmed during operation?

A rigid sigmoidoscopy may be performed to exclude rectal perforation. The cul-de-sac is first filled with irrigation fluid. As air is introduced through the sigmoidoscope into the rectum, in the presence of a perforation in the rectum, air bubbles will be seen in the cul-de-sac.

Alternatively, a Foley catheter may be introduced into the rectum; indigo carmine dye is then injected into the rectum through the catheter. If the dye escapes into the cul-de-sac, a perforated rectum is confirmed. A small perforation may be repaired with primary closure[1]. However, the decision on whether a primary closure or temporary colostomy/ileostomy is more appropriate in cases of rectal perforation should always be discussed and co-managed with a colorectal surgeon.

Outcome of various treatments for rectovaginal endometriosis

The outcome of laparoscopic treatment of rectovaginal endometriosis reported in the literature is summarized in Table 5.1. There are very few published data on the laparotomy approach to the management of rectovaginal endometriosis. The available data suggest encouraging results with good pain relief and cure for these patients[1,3,15]. Our own small series with the use of an open microsurgical approach also had very encouraging results. The recurrence of pelvic pain depends on the duration of follow-up and direct comparison between the series may not be appropriate.

Table 5.1 The outcome of laparoscopic and open microsurgery for rectovaginal endometriosis

Authors	Donnez et al.[3]	Nezhat et al.[1]	Reich et al.[15]	Sheffield series
Type of surgery	Laparoscopic surgery	Laparoscopic surgery	Laparoscopic surgery	Open microsurgery
Patients (n)	231	185	100	17
Duration of operation (range in minutes)	45–120	55–245	40–475	120–360
Duration of hospital stay (range in days)	2–5	1–4	1–2	4–14
Complication rate (%)*	3.5	6.5	4	5.8
Recurrence of pelvic pain (%)	1.5	6.0	11	12

*Complication rate includes hemorrhage, ureteric/bowel injury and compartment syndrome

Hormone replacement therapy

Hormone replacement therapy (HRT) may be required in young patients who have had excision of rectovaginal endometriosis as well as total abdominal hysterectomy. In theory, any residual endometriotic lesions regress in a hypoestrogenic state but may be reactivated in response to estrogenic stimulation. Various studies have reported conflicting results on the use of HRT following oophorectomy as part of the surgical management of endometriosis[21–25]. As progestogens inhibit the proliferation of endometrium, a continuous combined HRT preparation may be of theoretical advantage[22].

CONCLUSION

The diagnosis of rectovaginal endometriosis should be considered in patients with chronic pelvic pain associated with significant dyspareunia/dysmenorrhea. As the diagnosis is made mainly by clinical examination, a combined vaginal and rectal examination should be performed specifically looking for the signs of this condition, preferably at the time of menstruation. These patients should be managed by gynecologists with a special interest in rectovaginal endometriosis and with the assistance of a bowel surgeon. The principle of treatment is complete excision of the endometriotic and scar tissues. The gynecologist's familiarity and experience with these techniques will determine the choice of laparotomy or laparoscopy.

REFERENCES

1. Nezhat F, Nezhat C, Pennington E. Laparoscopic proctectomy for infiltrating endometriosis of the rectum. Fertil Steril 1992; 57: 1129–32.

2. Leiman G, Markowitz S, Veiga-Ferreira MM, et al. Endometriosis of the rectovaginal septum: diagnosis by fine needle aspiration cytology. Acta Cytol 1986; 30: 313–16.

3. Donnez J, Nisolle M, Casanas-Roux F, et al. Rectovaginal septum, endometriosis or adenomyosis: laparoscopic management in a series of 231 patients. Hum Reprod 1995; 10: 630–5.

4. Koninckx PR, Martin D. Treatment of deeply infiltrating endometriosis. Curr Opin Obstet Gynecol 1994; 6: 231–41.

5. American Fertility Society. Revised American Fertility Society classification of endometriosis. Fertil Steril 1985; 43: 351–2.

6. Brooks JJ, Wheeler JE. Malignancy arising in extragonadal endometriosis: a case report and summary of the world literature. Cancer 1977; 40: 3065–73.

7. Bailey HR, Ott MT, Hartendorp P. Aggressive surgical management for advanced colorectal endometriosis. Dis Colon Rectum 1985; 37: 747–53.

8. March CM, Israel R. Rectovaginal endometriosis: an isolated enigma. Am J Obstet Gynecol 1976; 125: 274–5.

9. Fedele L, Bianchi S, Portuese A, et al. Transrectal ultrasonography in the assessment of rectovaginal endometriosis. Obstet Gynecol 1998; 91: 444–8.

10. Singhal V, Li TC, Cooke ID. An analysis of factors influencing the outcome of 232 consecutive tubal microsurgery cases. Br J Obstet Gynaecol 1991; 98: 628–36.

11. Gomel V. From microsurgery to laparoscopic surgery: a progress. Fertil Steril 1995; 63: 464–8.

12.   Garry R. Laparoscopic excision of endometriosis: the treatment of choice? Br J Obstet Gynaecol 1997; 104: 513–15.

13.   Martin DC. Laparoscopic and vaginal colpotomy for the excision of infiltrating cul-de-sac endometriosis. J Reprod Med 1988; 33: 806–7.

14.   Redwine DB. Conservative laparoscopic excision of endometriosis by sharp dissection: life table analysis of reoperation and persistent or recurrent disease. Fertil Steril 1991; 56: 628–34.

15.   Reich H, McGlynn F, Slavat J. Laparoscopic treatment of cul-de-sac obliteration secondary to rectocervical deep fibrotic endometriosis. J Reprod Med 1991; 36: 516–22.

16.   Wood C, Maher P. Peritoneal surgery in the treatment of endometriosis – excision or thermal ablation? Aust NZ J Obstet Gynaecol 1996; 36: 190–7.

17.   Redwine DB, Perez JJ. Pelvic pain syndrome: endometriosis and midline dysmenorrhoea. In Arregui ME, Fitzgibbons RJ, Katkhouda N, et al., eds. Principles of Laparoscopic Surgery – Basic and Advanced Techniques. New York: Springer Verlag, 1995: 545–58.

18.   Nezhat C, Nezhat FR. Safer laser endoscopic excision or vaporisation of peritoneal endometriosis. Fertil Steril 1989; 52: 149–51.

19.   Dorsey JH. Indications and general techniques for lasers in advanced operative laparoscopy. Obstet Gynecol Clin North Am 1991; 18: 555–67.

20.   Busacca M, Bianchi S, Agnoli B, et al. Follow up of laparoscopic treatment of Stage III–IV endometriosis. J Am Assoc Gynecol Laparosc 1999; 6: 55–8.

21.   Langmade CF. Pelvic endometriosis and ureteral obstruction. Am J Obstet Gynecol 1975; 1: 463–9.

22.   Coronado C, Franklin RR, Lotze EC. Surgical treatment of symptomatic colorectal endometriosis. Fertil Steril 1990; 53: 411–16.

23.   Lam AM, French M, Charnock FM. Bilateral ureteric obstruction due to recurrent endometriosis associated with hormone replacement therapy. Aust NZ J Obstet Gynaecol 1992; 3: 83–4.

24.   Redwine DB. Endometriosis persisting after castration: clinical characteristics and result of surgical management. Obstet Gynecol 1994; 83: 405–13.

25.   Brough RJ, O'Flynn K. Recurrent pelvic endometriosis and bilateral ureteric obstruction associated with hormone replacement therapy. Br Med J 1996; 31: 11–12.

6 | Ovarian remnant syndrome

William L Ledger

INTRODUCTION

Ovarian remnant syndrome (ORS) is poorly understood, under-researched and infrequently discussed. A recent 1000-page textbook devoted entirely to gynecology[1] gave a description of the syndrome in only 10 lines. Although a Medline search using the terms 'ovary or ovarian' and 'remnant' (4 April 2004) revealed 105 references, about half discuss the syndrome in dogs and cats (an apparently well-known consequence of 'spaying'[2]) and the remainder are mostly individual case reports. ORS was first described in the 1960s[3], and by 1989, 36 cases had been published[4].

The syndrome describes postsurgical pain occurring after oophorectomy. A remnant of ovarian tissue remains endocrinologically active, with continuing folliculogenesis and production of estradiol. It is apparent that small remnant volumes of ovarian tissue may contain numerous primordial follicles, which can undergo follicle recruitment, selection and establishment of dominance, and produce large antral follicles that can ovulate and generate a corpus luteum – in other words continuing to follow the normal ovarian cycle. Experiments in cynomolgus monkeys[5] have shown that removal of the whole of one ovary and 90% of the other leads to only temporary cessation of ovarian cycles. Menstrual cycles rapidly resumed and histology of the ovarian remnant tissue revealed many small follicles. Of a group of monkeys that underwent 95% oophorectomy, two of six continued with regular cycles over a year later. Small fragments of ovarian tissue are clearly capable of causing great mischief.

PATHOGENESIS

The common presenting symptom of ORS is pain. The ovarian tissue is trapped within surgical adhesions and scarring, such that the cyclical enlargement of the ovarian remnant leads to pressure on adjacent pelvic and retroperitoneal structures, including the posterior vagina, rectum, bladder and ureter. There may also be cyclical production of pain-mediating molecules. One or both of these mechanisms leads to symptoms of lateralized intermittent discomfort and pain, back pain, 'irritable bowel syndrome' and dyspareunia. Other, rare presentations include ureteric obstruction and acute urinary retention[4,6,7], asymptomatic inclusion cysts seen on ultrasound[6] and cancer within the remnant tissue[8–12]. In most cases, there will be a history of complicated hysterectomy and oophorectomy, with the majority of patients having had initial surgery for endometriosis[13,14], pelvic inflammatory disease or inflammatory bowel disease[15]. Ovarian endometriomas are frequently adherent to adjacent structures, including those on the pelvic side wall. Surgeons are sensibly careful to avoid damage to the ureter, the course of which may run beneath or even into the wall of an endometrioma. It is therefore not surprising that ovarian remnant tissue may occasionally be left behind in such circumstances, discretion being preferable to valor in pelvic side-wall surgery. There may also be a history of several other surgical procedures carried out in an attempt to treat chronic pelvic pain, with either failure to identify the ovarian remnant or to treat it satisfactorily.

Although the paucity of literature on ORS precludes accurate estimation of its incidence, diagnosis seems to be becoming more frequent with widespread access to transvaginal ultrasound and laparoscopy. One series of 119 women who had laparoscopy to investigate pelvic pain after hysterectomy and oophorectomy found ORS in 26 (18%) cases[16]. Women with chronic pelvic pain following hysterectomy and bilateral oophorectomy may be dismissed as having 'non-gynecological' pain. Perhaps an increased awareness of the possibility of ORS may have led to a greater willingness on the part of the gynecologist to look for this diagnosis in more recent times.

DIAGNOSIS

As ever, the most important contribution in reaching a diagnosis will come from the history of previous oophorectomy, probably carried out in difficult circumstances. Physical examination may reveal a pelvic mass, fixation of the vaginal vault or lateralized pain. Biochemical investigation may show a surprisingly low concentration of follicle-stimulating hormone in the serum of a woman who has had bilateral oophorectomy, and measurable concentrations of estradiol may also be detected. Transvaginal ultrasound may show cystic structures arising from trapped ovarian follicles, surrounded by a rim of solid tissue. There may also be 'pseudocysts' – fluid collections lying between leafs of adhesions. These may be septate and can mimic malignant cysts. Color Doppler studies may well reveal significant vascular supply to the remnant[6]. Magnetic resonance imaging and computed tomography may also be helpful in certain cases[15,17], and an intravenous urogram should be organized to delineate the course of the ureter and identify any stricture due to ORS[18].

A number of diagnostic tests have been described. A course of ovarian stimulation using clomifene citrate may result in the appearance of follicles on ultrasound, with rising estradiol concentration in serum. This approach may be useful if there have been multiple previous attempts at pelvic surgery leading to a complex appearance on ultrasound without stimulation[19], and may also facilitate identification and removal of the remnant at surgery[20]. Alternatively, a gonadotropin-releasing hormone (GnRH) agonist stimulation test, with detection of a 'flare' in concentrations of estradiol in the serum of women with chronic pelvic pain suspected of harboring an ovarian remnant, has also been described[21].

TREATMENT

Medical treatment of ORS using pituitary downregulation with a GnRH agonist may be helpful for decompression of an obstructed ureter or shrinkage of a large pelvic mass. Treatment with estrogens and gestagens has not been found to be helpful[18]. In any case, medical treatment can only be regarded at best as a short-term solution and surgery will be necessary in almost all cases.

The gynecologist contemplating surgery for resolution of ORS must be cognisant of the potential difficulties that may be encountered. These are related to the proximity of the pelvic side-wall structures, ureter and great vessel, to the ovarian pedicle. Postsurgical adhesions frequently tether the remnant to the side wall and a case approached some years after the primary procedure may well involve extensive retroperitoneal dissection due to infiltration of ovarian adhesions into the retroperitoneal space. Whether the surgical approach is by laparotomy or laparoscopy, certain basic principles apply to the prosecution of successful surgery, namely comprehensive preoperative investigation, meticulous surgical technique and involvement of appropriately skilled colleagues. Details of preoperative assessment are described above. Each case must be assessed individually as the volume and situation of the remnant, and the extent of symptoms, will vary. At the least, preoperative transvaginal ultrasound and intravenous urogram should be arranged, and close collaboration with a competent radiologist is essential. Given that surgical complications are likely to involve damage to the ureter, bowel or blood vessels, it is advisable also to be able to call upon the services of competent colleagues in urology and colorectal and vascular surgery. Our surgical approach to ORS in Sheffield frequently involves ureteric stenting at the start of the procedure, to facilitate identification of the course of the ureter. This allows more confident retroperitoneal dissection and increases the likelihood of complete excision of the remnant.

Whilst early reports describe excision of ovarian remnants at laparotomy, a laparoscopic approach has had increasing interest over the last 15 years. The general advantages of laparoscopic surgery have been well described elsewhere, but it may also be the case that laparoscopy, with magnification of the view of anatomical structures, gives a better view of the pelvic side wall than can be obtained at laparotomy. If there is a complex history of previous abdominal surgery it may be prudent to use an open laparoscopic approach, and these cases should not be attempted by inexperienced laparoscopic surgeons. However, a number of case series have documented the safety and efficacy of laparoscopy for surgery to ovarian remnants[22–25]. Others continue to advocate laparotomy as the safest approach[1]. In practice, gynecological surgeons in the 21st century should be familiar with both approaches, as obstetricians should be competent at both forceps and ventouse delivery. Cases can then be individualized according to their complexity.

COMPLICATIONS

Probably the most frequently encountered 'complication' of ovarian remnant surgery is failure to remove the complete remnant. Even small amounts of ovarian tissue can contain many thousands of primordial follicles and the surgeon must be meticulous in clearing the operative field of both ovarian and apparently fibrous tissue remnants. Again, surgical confidence can be increased by ureteric stenting in selected cases.

Preoperative counseling must include an appraisal of the risks of the procedure, including those of damage to the ureter or blood vessels necessitating the need for emergency surgery and prolonged recovery. It is not possible to give accurate estimates of the degree of risk in an individual case – the size, location and degree of adhesion of ovarian remnants vary considerably, and the world literature is too small to devise accurate risk estimates. A written record of the areas covered in preoperative counseling should be made.

CONCLUSIONS

The management of ORS in younger patients will require surgery in most cases. This surgery should be carried out in a recognized centre, by an experienced team with good interdisciplinary collaboration. Complete removal of the remnant should lead to the resolution of symptoms, although clearance can be complicated by adhesions and proximity to important structures. Perhaps most importantly, surgeons performing oophorectomy should take care to remove all ovarian tissue. This will obviously be more difficult in complex cases, but time spent during the primary procedure may well save much effort later.

REFERENCES

1. Stones RW. Chronic pelvic pain. In Shaw R, Soutter P, Stanton S, eds. Gynaecology. Edinburgh: Churchill Livingstone, 2003: 887.

2. Miller DM. Ovarian remnant syndrome in dogs and cats: 46 cases. J Vet Diagn Invest 1995; 7: 572–4.

3. Shemwell RE, Weed JC. Ovarian remnant syndrome. Obstet Gynecol 1970; 36: 299–303.

4. Bryce GM, Malone P. The ovarian remnant syndrome presenting with acute urinary retention. Postgrad Med J 1989; 65: 797–8.

5. Danforth Dr, Chillik CF, Hertz R, Hodgen GD. Effects of ovarian tissue reduction on the menstrual cycle: persistent normalcy after near-total oophorectomy. Biol Reprod 1989; 41: 355–60.

6. Fleischer AC, Taid D, Mayo J, et al. Sonographic features of ovarian remnants. J Ultrasound Med 1998; 17: 551–5.

7. Visentini E, Bondavalli C, Pegoraro C, et al. Ovarian remnant syndrome: a case report. Arch Ital Nefrol Androl 1990; 62: 69–71.

8.   Bruhwiler H, Luscher KP. Ovarian cancer in ovarian remnant syndrome. Geburtshilfe Frauenheilkd 1991; 51: 70–1.

9.   Buanga K, Escorza MCL, Garcia GL. Ovarian remnant syndrome. A case report of a malignancy. J Gynaecol Obstet Biol Reprod (Paris) 1992; 21: 769–72.

10. Elkins TE, Stocker RJ, Key D, et al. Surgery for ovarian remnant syndrome. Lessons learned from difficult cases. J Reprod Med 1994; 39: 446–8.

11. Hamid R, May D. Ovarian malignancy in remnant ovarian tissue. Int J Gynecol Obstet 1997; 58: 319–20.

12. Narayansingh G, Cumming G, Parkin D, Miller I. Ovarian cancer developing in the ovarian remnant syndrome. Aust NZ J Obstet Gynaecol 2000; 40: 221–3.

13. Nezhat CG, Seidman DS, Nezhat FR, et al. Ovarian remnant syndrome after laparoscopic oophorectomy. Fertil Steril 2000; 74: 1024–8.

14. Rana N, Rotman C, Hasson HM, et al. Ovarian remnant syndrome after laparoscopic hysterectomy and bilateral salpingo oophorectomy for severe pelvic endometriosis. Am Assoc Gynecol Laparosc 1996; 3: 423–6.

15. Pettit PD, Lee RA. Ovarian remnant syndrome: diagnostic dilemma and surgical challenge. Obstet Gynecol 1988; 71: 580–3.

16. Abu-Rafeh B, Vilos GA, Misra M. Frequency and laparoscopic management of ovarian remnant syndrome. J Am Assoc Gynecol Laparosc 2003; 10: 33–7.

17. Webb MJ. Ovarian remnant syndrome. Aust NZ J Obstet Gynaecol 1989; 29: 433–5.

18. Steege JF. Ovarian remnant syndrome. Obstet Gynecol 1987; 70: 64–7.

19. Orford VP, Kuhn RJ. Management of the ovarian remnant syndrome. Aust NZ J Obstet Gynaecol 1996; 36: 468–71.

20. Kaminski PF, Sorosky JI, Mandell MJ, et al. Clomiphene citrate stimulation as an adjunct in locating ovarian tissue in ovarian remnant syndrome. Obstet Gynecol 1990; 76: 924–6.

21. Scott RT, Beatse SN, Illions EH, Snyder RR. Use of the GnRH agonist stimulation test in the diagnosis of ovarian remnant syndrome. A report of three cases. J Reprod Med 1995; 40: 143–6.

22. Mahdavi A, Berker B, Nezhat C, et al. Laparoscopic management of ovarian remnant. Obstet Gynecol Clin North Am 2004; 31:593–7.

23. Kamprath S, Possover M, Schneider A. Description of a laparoscopic technique for treating patients with ovarian remnant syndrome. Fertil Steril 1997; 68: 663–7.

24. Dionisi HJ, Dionisi JE, Dionisi JM. Laparoscopic treatment of ovarian retention pathology. J Am Assoc Gynecol Laparosc 1996; (4 Suppl): S10.

25. Nezhat F, Nezhat C. Operative laparoscopy for the treatment of ovarian remnant syndrome. Fertil Steril 1992; 57: 1003–7.

7 Painful bladder syndrome

Sheilagh Reid, Derek Rosario

INTRODUCTION

Painful bladder syndrome (PBS) is characterized by suprapubic pain and storage lower urinary tract symptoms (LUTS) in the presence of normal urine on culture. In a subgroup of women, anterior vaginal or urethral pain may be present and indeed, predominate in a minority. In some patients, a definite etiological agent may be identified; however, in the majority no definite cause is found. Many such patients may have been labeled with chronic pelvic pain syndrome or interstitial cystitis (IC). These are conditions which are poorly defined and often mean different things to different clinicians, as well raising expectations in patients. In dealing with pelvic pain of uncertain origin, it is probably best to avoid such labeling until comprehensive evaluation has been carried out, which may include cystoscopy and laparoscopy. The principles of management are:

(1) To identify (or exclude) treatable causes of bladder/urethral pain;

(2) To provide a multidisciplinary and multimodality approach to pain management; and

(3) To provide information and support.

The involvement of pain specialists, behavioral therapists and patient groups is critical, but only when all possible treatable causes have been explored and excluded by thorough patient evaluation, preferably in a multidisciplinary setting.

ETIOLOGY

Etiological agents of LUTS and pelvic pain include radiation cystitis, cyclophosphamide cystitis and bladder cancer (most typically carcinoma *in situ*). It is imperative that malignancy is not overlooked in these patients. Flexible cystoscopy will reveal the majority of malignancies but it is still possible to overlook widespread carcinoma *in situ*. This typically presents with symptoms of 'cystitis' and a voiding pattern of frequent small-volume urinations – the so-called 'staccato bladder'. A frequency volume chart can be very useful to raise suspicion. For diagnosis it is necessary to perform rigid cystoscopy under general anesthetic to allow biopsies to be taken. The most common cause of LUTS and pelvic pain is infection. This is usually easy to diagnose with urinary microscopy. It is worth remembering that there are some microorganisms that are not easy to culture and that may be missed, so there can be a role for antimicrobial treatment in the presence of a negative culture.

The vast majority of non-infective cases, however, do not have a defined etiology and belong to a group of conditions known as pelvic pain syndrome. IC is the label most widely used although it can encompass a wide range of bladder problems. The bulk of this chapter will focus on interstitial cystitis.

PRESENTATION

The majority of sufferers are females in their childbearing years; however, it is becoming increasingly apparent that men with a label of chronic prostatitis often have very similar symptoms to many women with a diagnosis of PBS/IC. Both conditions are diagnoses of exclusion rather than inclusion. As such, IC has been described by the late Professor Tage Hald as a 'hole in the air' diagnosis[1]. This chapter will deal exclusively with adult female practice, concentrating on PBS/IC.

EPIDEMIOLOGY

The International Continence Society[2] defines PBS as 'the complaint of suprapubic pain related to bladder filling accompanied by other symptoms such as increased daytime and night time frequency in the absence of proven infection or other obvious pathology'. IC is the name often used for patients with PBS without a known cause. The International Continence Society reserves the diagnosis of IC for those patients with PBS who have typical cystoscopic and histological findings[2], but does not specify what these findings are. The condition was described originally by Skene in 1887[3], but it was Hunner (1915)[4] who reported on eight women with suprapubic pain frequency, nocturia and urgency, and provided the classic description of a bladder 'ulcer', given the name Hunner's ulcer. Some investigators subclassify IC into ulcerative (the minority of cases) and non-ulcerative (the majority of cases). This can be useful in practice as surgical intervention may be more effective in relieving symptoms in women with the ulcerative pattern than those without. This may merely be a reflection of disease severity and impact on quality of life rather than pointing to a specific diagnostic difference between the conditions.

Providing a definition whereby patients could be compared, with a view to diagnosis, treatments and outcomes, is difficult. In 1987, the National Institute of Diabetes and Digestive and Kidney Diseases (NIDDK) held a workshop to establish criteria for the diagnosis of IC. These criteria (Table 7.1) were not meant to define the disease but rather were supposed to be a research tool whereby patients could be appropriately entered into clinical trials[5]. The criteria were revised after a workshop in 1988 and published in a book[6] (Table 7.2). This has resulted in two rather dissimilar sets of NIDDK criteria, which has led to some confusion among clinicians.

Estimates of prevalence are based on population-based studies, the first of which was carried out in Finland[7]. In a population of approximately one million, the prevalence in women was 18.1 per 100 000. The annual incidence of new female cases was 1.2 per 100 000. Severe cases accounted for 10% of the total and approximately 10% of cases were described in men. Subsequent studies have reported a prevalence ranging from 10 per 100 000 to 60 per 100 000[8,9] with the female : male ratio consistently 10 : 1. The most recent data found a significantly higher rate, with at least 10% of the female medical students in the study having IC[10]. The wide variation in these studies outlines the problem of diagnosing and reporting PBS/IC. Table 7.3 outlines the reported prevalences and the method of data collection in these studies.

There is no known association of PBS/IC with malignancy, although malignancy must be excluded when making the initial diagnosis. Associated disorders include irritable bowel (30%)[11], fibromyalgia[12], inflammatory bowel disease[13], focal vulvitis[14], chronic urticaria[15] and Sjogren's syndrome[16].

PBS/IC is a chronic disorder that relapses and remits. There is a 50% incidence of temporary remission unrelated to therapy, with a mean duration of 8 months[17]. There is no evidence of a progressive increase in severity of symptoms in women managed conservatively over 4 years[18].

Table 7.1 NIDDK inclusion and exclusion criteria for interstitial cystitis, established at a workshop in 1987[5]

Inclusion criteria (two positive factors necessary for inclusion)	Exclusion criteria
Hunner's ulcer – automatic inclusion	< 18 years of age
Pain on bladder filling relieved by emptying	Benign or malignant bladder tumors
	Radiation cystitis
Pain (suprapubic, pelvic, urethral, vaginal or perineal)	Tuberculous cystitis
	Bacterial cystitis
Glomerulations on endoscopy	Vaginitis
Decreased bladder compliance on cystometrogram	Cyclophosphamide cystitis
	Symptomatic urethral diverticulum
	Uterine, cervical, vaginal or urethral cancer
	Active herpes
	Bladder or lower ureteric calculi
	Waking frequency < 5 times in 12 hours
	Nocturia < 2 times
	Symptoms relieved by antibiotics, urinary antiseptics, urinary analgesics (for example phenazopyridine hydrochloride)
	Duration < 12 months
	Involuntary bladder contractions (urodynamics)
	Capacity > 400 cc, absence of sensory urgency

NIDDK, National Institute of Diabetes and Digestive and Kidney Diseases

PATHOGENESIS

The pathogenesis of PBS/IC is not fully understood and is generally accepted to be multifactorial. The many studies to date show mast cell activation with neural, immune and endocrine components, and an alteration in the glycosaminoglycan (GAG)-rich mucus lining the bladder wall with increased epithelial permeability.

Animal models for the condition have been sought. The closest potential model is in cats – the so-called feline urologic syndrome – who experience

Table 7.2 Revised criteria after the 1988 workshop[6]

Inclusion criteria	Exclusion criteria
Either glomerulations on cystoscopic examination or a classic Hunner's ulcer	Bladder capacity greater than 350 ml on awake cystometry using either gas or liquid as a filling medium
Either pain associated with the bladder or urinary urgency	Absence of an intense urge to void with the bladder filled to 100 ml with gas or 150 ml with water during cystometry, using a fill rate of 30–100 ml/min
	The demonstration of phasic involuntary bladder contractions on cystometry using the fill rate described
	Duration of symptoms less than 9 months
	Absence of nocturia
	Symptoms relieved by antibiotics, urinary antiseptics, urinary analgesics (for example phenazopyridine hydrochloride)
	A frequency of urination while awake of less than 8 times a day
	A diagnosis of bacterial cystitis or prostatitis within a 3-month period
	Active herpes
	Bladder or lower ureteral calculi
	Radiation cystitis
	Tuberculous cystitis
	Bacterial cystitis
	Vaginitis
	Cyclophosphamide cystitis
	Uterine, cervical, vaginal or urethral cancer
	Benign or malignant bladder tumors
	Age < 18 years

frequency, urgency, pain and bladder inflammation in the presence of sterile urine. Glomerulations have been found in the bladder of some of these cats. A decrease in the expression of a GAG has also been found in these cats[19–21]. Whether this model will provide useful information remains to be seen.

Table 7.3 Incidence and prevalence of painful bladder syndrome/interstitial cystitis (IC) reported in the literature

Study	Incidence	Prevalence	How obtained?
Oravisto 1975[7]	1.2/100 000 per year	18.1/100 000	Found 'all' cases of IC in Helsinki and related them to the total population
Bade 1995[8]		8–16/100 000	Questionnaire completed by urologists
Curhan 1999[9]		52–67/100 000	Asked via a mailed questionnaire if they had IC
Parsons 2004[10]		10% documented and 36% probable	Female members of a single class of medical students using a validated questionnaire; those scoring high underwent clinical evaluation including a potassium sensitivity test

In a healthy bladder, the transitional epithelium is relatively impermeable. The main barrier lies in the nature of the uroplakins expressed on the umbrella cells of the urothelial lining. There is in addition to this a GAG layer composed of proteoglycans (rich in GAG) and glycoproteins[22,23]. The function of the GAG layer is not well understood, but it may have a role in preventing constituents of urine from coming into contact with the urothelium. The GAG layer is produced by the urothelial cells. Any deficiency of the GAG layer therefore implies an underlying abnormality in these cells. Studies have found epithelial dysfunction causing increased permeability in patients with IC, compared with those with normal bladders, with permeability being greatest in those with the worst disease[24]. This same dysfunction has been found in bladders of cats with feline urologic syndrome[19]. The concept of lower urinary dysfunctional epithelium as a cause of urinary urgency and/or pelvic pain, including dyspareunia, in younger patients (less than 55 years) is strongly put forward by Parsons[25]. This report proposes that potassium is present in the urine at concentrations that are toxic to muscles and nerves. In the normal bladder, potassium has no effect because of the protective mucus, but when the epithelial permeability is compromised, it can diffuse into the interstitium and depolarize nerves and muscle, leading to tissue injury and destruction. The same mechanism would explain the symptoms from acute bacterial cystitis, radiation cystitis or carcinoma *in situ*, where patients also have epithelial injury, except in these cases (unlike IC) the cause of the epithelial damage is known. Parsons tested this concept using the potassium sensitivity test (PST). This involved instilling potassium chloride into the bladder; patients with normal bladders had no response to this, in contrast to those with abnormally permeable epithelium who experienced symptoms of urgency and/or pain. Patients with urethral syndrome and prostatitis were found to have similar rates of response to the PST as those with IC, leading to the conclusion that they are part of the same pathological process. Parsons has supported the use of this test for examining symptomatic populations and, although this is not in general usage, the concept provides valuable insight into IC. However, Yilmaz[26] used this test on a group of men with IC/chronic pain syndrome and found no statistical difference between healthy men and those affected, although pain and urgency were increased after instillation.

Mast cells have been found to be associated with IC. A number of reports exist citing mastocytosis as either causative or as a pathognomonic marker[27–29]. Bladder biopsies from IC patients have an increased number of activated mast cells[30]. Mast cells are located in the bladder close to blood vessels, nerves and detrusor muscle[31]. They release histamine as well as other components, and this can cause tissue pain, hyperemia and fibrosis, which are all found in the IC bladder. The many studies that have examined mast cells in IC have strongly suggested that activated mast cells play a central, though not primary, role in the disease, although exactly what activates them is unclear[32].

Neurogenic inflammation as a cause of IC also has a body of evidence. Activation of sensory nerves can cause inflammation through release of neuropeptides such as substance P. Neuropeptides can cause degranulation of mast cells[33]. An increase in nerve fibers within the suburothelium and detrusor muscle in ulcerative IC has been found[34]. A defective GAG layer and the penetrating products from urine could lead to sensitization of neurons to secrete neuropeptides with activation of mast cells.

There is also evidence that autoimmune factors may have a role to play. Oravisto concluded that the chronic course of the disease, absence of infection and occurrence of antinuclear antibodies provided strong evidence of autoimmunity[35]. There has been much written since but the overall role of autoimmunity is controversial[36].

The overriding preponderance of IC in females has led to speculation about hormonal involvement in the disease. Indeed, bladder mast cells express high-affinity estrogen receptors and there are a higher number of these cells in patients with IC than controls[36]. There is not, however, any good evidence to take this speculation further.

Although the mechanisms described would explain much about the disease they do little to enlighten us on possible etiology. The role of infection and/or antibiotic treatment has been investigated. Most patients with IC have initially been thought to have infections and, in some cases, to have received many courses of antibiotics. There is also the fact that the onset of the disease is often very sudden, with many patients remembering the day their symptoms commenced. Attempts to treat the disease with intensive antibiotics have been tried but a prospective, double-blind randomized controlled trial showed only minimal improvement in some patients in the active arm and concluded that intensive antibiotic treatment was not the answer[37]. However, intensive searching for an infective cause, including the use of DNA and RNA probes, has so far proved unsuccessful[38–40]. There is a theory, however, that bacterial cystitis may be the first step in a cascade of bladder wall damage with low-level inflammatory response[41]. Despite the lack of evidence a recent study examined the treatment of women with doxycycline[42]. The authors noted that many women with urinary symptoms and pain, but with no conclusive evidence of infection, had trigonal leukoplakia, thought to be a sign of chronic infection. Doxycycline is a broad-spectrum antibiotic effective against organisms not routinely detected by urinary cultures, such as *Chlamydia trachomatis*, *Ureaplasma urealyticum* and *Mycoplasma genitalium*. Critically, in this study the sexual partner was also fully treated. More than two-thirds of the women (71%) were either symptom-free or had a subjective decrease in their symptoms after treatment.

In summary, the etiology of IC remains unclear. There appears to be an alteration in the GAG-rich mucus lining the bladder wall, with an increase in epithelial permeability. A defect in this protective GAG layer results in leakage of noxious substances and mast cell-mediated neuroinflammation, irritating the deeper layers. This may induce stimulation of neural pathways, resulting in pelvic floor pain and spasm, and sensitize neurons to secrete neurotransmittors that can further activate mast cells[43] (Figure 7.1).

PATIENT ASSESSMENT

A very apt description of a patient suffering from severe IC was provided by Bourque in 1951: 'we have all met at one time or another patients who suffer chronically from their bladder, and we mean the ones who are distressed, not only periodically but constantly, having to urinate often at all moments of the day or night and suffering pains every time they void. We all know how these miserable patients are unhappy, and how those distressing bladder symptoms get finally to influence their general state of health, physically at first and mentally after a while'[44].

Apart from pelvic pain, urinary symptoms can be of varying degrees. The predominant symptoms are storage in nature, mainly frequency and urgency. Quantifying frequency is difficult, with normal being seven to eight times in 24 hours, but this number will be altered by drinking habits and body temperature[45]. Frequency volume charts detailing all input are very helpful both to the clinician and to the patient, who often has surprisingly little appreciation of the association between insensible fluid intake (food, etc.) and output. Nocturia can cause significant sleep disturbance. Symptom indices show a significant impact of IC on a sufferer's quality of life when compared with controls[46]. Urinary incontinence is unusual although stress urinary incontinence may coexist. Indeed, the

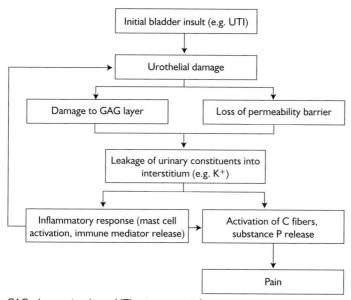

GAG, glycosaminoglycan; UTI, urinary tract infection

Figure 7.1 Proposed mechanisms in the pathogenesis of painful bladder syndrome/interstitial cystitis

presence of urinary incontinence should alert the clinician to the likely existence of an alternative diagnosis.

Pelvic pain is an essential component and may be insidious with intermittent flare cycles[47]. Pain can be localized in the perineum, labia or vagina causing female patients to present to gynecologists and undergo gynecological investigations, diverting attention from bladder problems. Dyspareunia may be a presenting symptom with patients presenting to gynecologists with deep genital pain associated with intercourse. Pain can also be localized to the rectum. Traditionally, the pain is suprapubic, increases on bladder filling and is relieved by bladder emptying. There are no criteria for the location of the pain, its severity or its character, except that it must be chronic in nature and have no other cause[45].

Initial patient assessment should aim to exclude known causes of the patient's problem; for example, noting a history of genitourinary infection, previous surgery, pelvic radiation or cyclophosphamide treatment. A history of hematuria always necessitates a full hematuria screen. Abdominal examination is likely to reveal suprapubic tenderness. Pelvic examination is essential. Vaginal examination, paying particular attention to the presence of a discharge, urethral palpation (an anterior wall mass or induration signifying a urethral diverticulum) and exclusion of gynecological malignancy, is necessary. However, it is often uncomfortable and may even be impossible. Digital rectal examination is a valuable adjunct in such cases.

Urine dipstick analysis should be performed at the time of initial assessment and any positive results should be sent for microscopy and culture analysis to exclude urinary tract infection. Patients with microscopic or macroscopic hematuria need full urological evaluation to exclude both lower and upper tract urological tumors. Any suspicion of genitourinary infection necessitates endocervical and urethral swabs placed in appropriate transport medium for the diagnosis of gonorrhoea and *Chlamydia*.

The next stage of assessment is rigid cystoscopy, which should be carried out under a light general anesthetic[36]. Some clinicians advocate flexible cystoscopy under local anesthetic as a less invasive option. Although this may be necessary in a very unfit patient, the discomfort associated with the procedure in such cases reduces its diagnostic value and causes unnecessary suffering to the patient. Furthermore, rigid cystoscopy under anesthesia allows a thorough pelvic examination, and the taking of adequate bladder biopsies, and provides an opportunity for a short hydrostatic distension, which has both diagnostic and potential therapeutic value.

Cystodistension is carried out as follows. A degree of Trendelenburg (head-down) tilt is helpful. Initial pelvic examination is carried out and, following this, the urethra is massaged and the presence or absence of discharge noted and swabs taken. The urethra is calibrated and dilated to 30 Ch. This allows diagnosis of urethral stenosis and easy introduction of the rigid cystoscope. A thorough cystoscopy is carried out starting with inspection of the trigone and ureteric orifices. Vaginal type squamous metaplasia is often present over the trigone and is thought to be of no clinical significance. The bladder is inspected in segments using the trigone and air bubble at the dome as the two poles. The degree of hyperemia, trabeculation and state of the mucosa are carefully assessed. Carcinoma *in situ* often appears as a red patch. Following initial cystoscopy, the bladder is hydrodistended to 80–100 cm with normal saline for 3 minutes[48]. The volume of water instilled varies between patients. The bag of normal saline should be 80–100 cm vertically above the urethra and the bladder should be filled until filling stops (Figure 7.2). A rise and fall of the level in the chamber will be seen at this point with the patient's breathing. Some patients develop tachycardia and tachypnea, which is usually a sign of more severe disease. Laryngospasm may occur and sometimes necessitates immediate bladder emptying. After the period of hydrodistension (3 minutes) the bladder is then drained, with bladder capacity and color of the effluent noted. The terminal portion may be blood-stained. Second-look cystoscopy is then performed. The presence of punctate petechial hemorrhages, known as glomerulations, is the main feature (Figure 7.3). However, not all patients with symptoms of PBS have glomerulations[49,50] and not all patients with glomerulations have symptoms of PBS[51]. Therefore, glomerulations are not specific for PBS and are only significant if found associated with symptoms of pain, urgency and frequency. The presence of a Hunner's ulcer (red mucosa with small vessels radiating to a central pale scar) is more consistently associated with pain and urgency[50] but the perception of what a Hunner's ulcer is varies hugely.

The role of biopsy and histopathology is primarily to exclude other diseases. There are no pathological changes that are pathognomonic for PBS although certain changes – severe lamina propria fibrosis[52], severe inflammation[52], detrusor fibrosis[52,53], mast cell infiltration[52,53] and detrusor myopathy[54] – correlate with a poorer clinical outcome.

Sufficient information can be gleaned from non-invasive urodynamics (frequency volume chart, uroflowmetry and residual urine estimation) to make cystometry unnecessary in the majority of patients. There is a role for formal

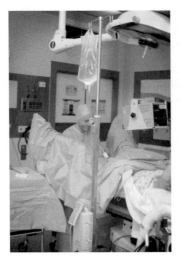 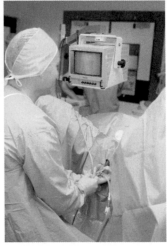

Cystoscopy is performed and the bag of irrigation fluid is placed 80 cm above the pubic symphysis of the patient. Filling continues until it stops spontaneously

The bladder is distended for 3 minutes with the surgeon's fingers compressing the urethra to prevent leakage of fluid around the cystoscope

Figure 7.2 Performance of cystodistension

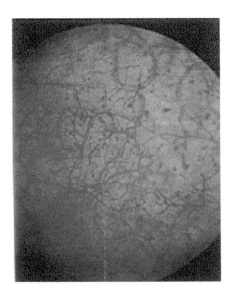

Figure 7.3 Cystoscopic appearance of glomerulations post-cystodistension

urodynamics in patients in whom incontinence is a significant problem. Overactive detrusor has been found in 14% of patients in the Interstitial Cystitis Data Base Study[55]. However, overactive bladder is found in a similar proportion of asymptomatic volunteers, hence the significance of this is uncertain. In our experience, the presence of significant incontinence usually signifies another diagnosis. Magnetic resonance imaging is a useful investigation if a urethral diverticulum is suspected (Figure 7.4). There may be an indication for laparoscopy for patients with chronic pelvic pain if there is dyspareunia or dysmenorrhea, to rule out endometriosis and other such conditions.

MANAGEMENT OF PBS

The management of PBS is multidisciplinary. The best that treatments can offer is symptomatic improvement. There are many reports on the effects of diet on symptoms; however, clinical data are lacking. Management of the disease requires a multidisciplinary approach, with drug intervention being just one of the modalities. As the condition remits and relapses spontaneously, the results of short-term trials indicating therapeutic benefit are difficult to interpret. Treatments can be broken down into conservative and surgical, with conservative measures

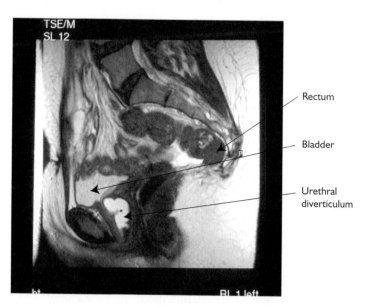

Figure 7.4   Magnetic resonance imaging of urethral diverticulum

being further subdivided into general strategies (including pain management, alternative therapies and psychological support) and specific disease-modifying interventions (such as immune modulation, neuromodulation and GAG layer replacement).

Conservative management – general measures

Management of pain

The use of simple analgesia (paracetamol, non-steroidal analgesics and mild opiates) is generally unhelpful in our experience but worth trying in the initial phases. Strong opiate analgesia is also not particularly helpful except at high doses, when the incidence of adverse events becomes a problem, and is generally best avoided because of problems with tolerance and dependency. Other treatments for neuropathic pain, such as gabapentin, have been used with some success[56].

Antidepressants

Tricyclic antidepressants, particularly amitriptyline, have for a long time been a mainstay of treatment for the pain component of PBS. A recent (and the only) randomized controlled trial using up to 100 mg of amitriptyline daily confirmed improvements in pain and urgency, with a statistically significant improvement in symptom score[57].

Antimicrobials

The use of antibiotics has been discussed in the earlier section on pathogenesis. There is no proven role in the absence of infection except for the use of doxycycline[42]. In the study by Burkhard et al. doxycycline was used at 100 mg twice daily for 2 weeks followed by 100 mg daily for 2 weeks[42]. To remove the vaginal potential to be a reservoir for infection, vaginal tablets (hexetidine or ciclopiroxolamine; once daily for 10 days) were also used and, crucially, the patients' sexual partners were treated with doxycycline 100 mg twice daily for 2 weeks. More than two-thirds had an improvement in symptoms after treatment.

Psychological support

Psychological support is one of the mainstays of long-term patient management and patients should be encouraged to contact one of the support groups. The Cystitis and Overactive Bladder Foundation has many local groups. The clinical nurse specialist has a very important role to play in this area.

Conservative management – disease-modifying drugs

There is little or no level I evidence for the use of drugs, either intravesically or orally, in the management of PBS/IC. Randomized controlled trials are few in number, preventing a meta-analysis, and have tended to include only a small number of patients. Much of the evidence, therefore, is experiential and based on an understanding of what the underlying pathology might be (e.g. GAG layer damage).

Mucosal surface protection

There is evidence that alteration in the GAG-rich mucus lining the bladder wall, with increased epithelial permeability, is a major factor in PBS. It is therefore logical that treatments should be targeted at mucosal surface protection[58]. Agents used in this manner include intravesical and subcutaneous heparin[59,60], intravesical hyaluronic acid (Cystistat)[61,62] and the heparin analog pentosan polysulfate (PPS; Elmiron).

PPS is used orally at a dose of 100 mg three times a day[63]. Several studies have been published on this drug, including randomized controlled trials[64–67]. These have shown a modest or no effect on symptoms but have confirmed that PPS is well tolerated with few side-effects. Efficacy has been reported in only about 30% of those using it long term[68], and symptomatic improvement takes 3–6 months.

Intravesical hyaluronic acid (Cystistat) has gained popularity, and patients with refractory IC have been described as having a 'gratifying' response to treatment, with no significant toxicity[62]. Anecdotally, Cystistat is more effective for the painful element than for urinary frequency. However, there is no conclusive evidence of subjective or objective improvement in patients from randomized controlled trials for this expensive drug that requires intensive input. Cystistat is given as an initial course of six instillations over 12 weeks. Four are given at weekly intervals and then a further two every 4 weeks. If the treatment is tolerated the interval can be increased to 6, 8 and 12 weeks; if the patient is well the treatment can then be stopped. A significant proportion of patients require maintenance treatment with instillations every 6–12 weeks. A few patients revert to two weekly treatments for short intervals during 'flares'. The dose is 40 mg of sodium hyaluronate (Cystistat) in 50 ml of saline and the patients are advised to hold it for at least 30 minutes before voiding.

Reduction of the inflammatory component

There is some evidence that mast cells are activated in PBS, causing pain and releasing inflammatory mediators[69]; antihistamines are used to treat this. The H1 blocker hydroxyzine blocks neuronal activation of mast cells[70]. Doses up to 25 mg in the morning and 50 mg at night have been used with some success although a blinded placebo-controlled trial has not been performed[69]. The most important side-effect of this drug is drowsiness and it may affect a patient's ability to drive or perform their job if given during the day. H2 blockers have also been used with some success (cimetidine 200 mg tds)[71] although the rationale for this is unclear. Other treatment regimes that have been tried are montelukast (a leukotriene-D4 receptor antagonist)[72], l-arginine[73], suplatast tosilate (IPD-1151T)[74], methotrexate[75] and cyclosporine[76]. None of these treatments have been shown to have significant effects in randomized controlled trials, although montelukast[72] shows promise and results of future trials are awaited.

Intravesical dimethylsulfoxide (DMSO) is an industrial solvent that has been used in the treatment of IC. It is administered via urethral catheter into the bladder; 50 ml of a 50% solution is retained for 15 minutes and then voided, every 1–2 weeks for four to eight treatments. Its mechanism of action may be due to depletion of substance P from the bladder wall and mast cell degranulation[77]. DMSO is associated with garlic-like breath for up to 2 days. Bladder spasm and hypersensitivity may occur and patients need ophthalmic, renal and hepatic assessment every 6 months. Response rates have been reported as 50–70% symptomatic improvement with 35–40% relapse that is generally responsive to further treatments[78]. Although a number of patients have remained on maintenance DMSO without any problem, DMSO remains an unlicensed treatment for this condition. With the advent of less toxic therapies, there is little justification for commencing newly diagnosed women with PBS on DMSO except under exceptional circumstances.

Conservative management – physical therapy

The rationale for the use of physical therapy in this condition is the theory that some pelvic pain may be caused either primarily or secondarily by myofascial tension. Therefore biofeedback and soft tissue massage causing muscle relaxation in the pelvic floor would help with symptoms. A recent study examined the use of the Thiele massage (transvaginal manual massage to the pelvic floor musculature) in 21 patients; treatment twice a week for 5 weeks showed some improvement in symptoms[79].

Conservative management – alternative therapies

The literature is surprisingly scant on the use of alternative therapies in PBS; since PBS is a chronic condition with relapses and remissions, such therapies should produce good results. Both yoga[80] and hypnosis[81] have been used with some reported success. The use of transcutaneous nerve stimulation of the posterior tibial nerve and the use of acupuncture were examined in a prospective study[82], although only a very limited effect was observed in patients with IC. However, because management of this disease relies heavily on patient empowerment and the ability to deal with their symptoms, physicians should be open to the potential benefits of alternative therapies.

Conservative management – neuromodulation

There is some evidence that patients refractory to other treatments for IC will respond to the use of sacral nerve stimulation. Permanent implantation of a neurogenerator[83] and percutaneous nerve root stimulation[84] have both been shown to produce symptomatic improvement.

Conservative management – immunomodulation

Immune responses have been suggested as playing a role in mucosal damage associated with PBS. Intravesical bacilli Calmette-Guerin, usually used as a treatment for carcinoma *in situ*, has been administered with some success to patients with PBS. Initially this treatment was given mistakenly in a misdiagnosis of carcinoma *in situ* but a subsequent small randomized controlled trial showed a significant sustained response in 60% of patients vs. 27% of controls[85]. More recently, a case has been reported in which a woman treated with anti-IgE therapy (omalizumab) for asthma and allergic symptoms was found to have complete symptomatic and cystoscopic resolution of previously ongoing IC[86].

Surgical intervention

The performance of bladder distension has been discussed in the earlier section on patient assessment. Bladder distension is used both in diagnosis and treatment with some patients experiencing improvement in symptoms commencing 2–3 weeks after the procedure and lasting for more than a year (60% improvement reported at 6 months)[87]. Historically it was performed for long periods of time with reported benefits (up to 3 hours)[88]. However, there is a potential for bladder rupture, particularly in patients with more severe IC, and some evidence to show that it gives no benefit over shorter distension times (minutes)[89]. Prolonged hydrodistension is therefore no longer recommended.

Patients who are considered for major surgery are the exceptions and all other avenues should have been explored prior to this. Surgery should only be carried out by urological surgeons specializing in this form of surgery. Bladder augmentation, supratrigonal cystectomy, subtrigonal cystectomy with orthotopic reconstruction, total cystectomy and urinary diversions are potential surgical options. In a supratrigonal cystectomy, the bladder is excised above the insertion of the ureters with sparing of the ureteric orifices and trigone. In a subtrigonal cystectomy the ureteric orifices and trigone are excised, with reimplantation of the ureters into the bowel segment forming the neo-bladder. In both cases, the bladder neck and urethra are left intact with preservation of the neurovascular bundles to the urethra. Patient selection is critical to success, with patients being able and willing to perform intermittent self-catheterization. The presence of urethral hypersensitivity, which often accompanies PBS, may make self-catheterization uncomfortable, in which case a Mitrofanoff procedure to provide an alternative catheterizable port can be carried out. Total cystectomy includes urethral excision and requires the formation of a urinary diversion. Results from surgery are not widely reported. Van Ophoven reported on 18 women undergoing supratrigonal cystectomy and orthotopic bladder reconstruction; 14 women (78%) were symptom-free at 5 years and four required catheterization[90]. A report on subtrigonal cystectomy with orthotopic bladder reconstruction showed that 82% of patients (14 of 17) were symptom-free at 5 years[91]. There is little evidence to support the choice between supratrigonal and total cystectomy. Anecdotally there is less retention with supratrigonal excision but a higher chance of ongoing symptoms if the trigone is left *in situ*. Patients opting to undergo a urinary diversion can either have a continent diversion or an ileal conduit. High patient motivation is required for the former. A urinary diversion without cystectomy is not advised as the patient will experience ongoing pelvic pain. Persistent pelvic pain despite cystectomy has been described.

Promising future treatments

Suplatast tosilate (IPD-1151T) is an oral medication that suppresses cytokine production in helper T cells, immunoglobulin E synthesis, chemical mediator release from mast cells and eosinophil recruitment. Early studies have shown improvements in urgency, frequency and pain in women with non-ulcerative IC[74].

Vanilloids are compounds that activate vanilloid receptors. They are thought to act by desensitizing C fibers, therefore stopping pain perception whatever the cause. Intravesical capsaicin and resiniferatoxin (a more potent capsaicin analog) have both been studied in randomized, placebo-controlled trials, showing symptom improvement[92,93]. Higher doses of these drugs, however, can produce retention.

Botulinum toxin works by inhibiting the release of acetylcholine. It has begun to be used to treat bladder problems. It is used by submucosal injection via a cystoscope into 20–30 sites in the trigone. A small study (13 patients) has been reported on its use in IC, showing both symptomatic and urodynamic improvement[94].

Immunotherapy has already been discussed and represents a promising route for further study.

The use of gene therapy in IC remains an exciting prospect for the future[58]. Specific targeting of treatment will require a better understanding of the factors involved in the etiology and promotion of the pain associated with PBS.

Figure 7.5 summarizes the overall management of patients with PBS.

CONCLUSIONS

PBS is a significant problem in terms of prevalence and impact on quality of life. It is not a well-defined condition, with diagnosis relying heavily on exclusion of other pathologies. The vast majority of patients can be managed conservatively and patient education, empowerment and support remain the mainstay of management.

Response to treatment is unpredictable and the true impact of interventions on symptoms, in a condition characterized by remissions, is difficult to assess. Having said that, the majority of patients respond to conservative management, with very few requiring major surgical intervention. The number of options

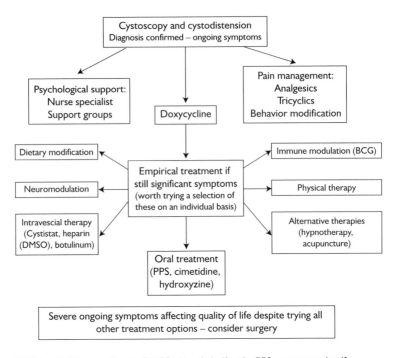

BCG, bacilli Calmette-Guerin; DMSO, dimethylsulfoxide; PPS, pentosanpolysulfate

Figure 7.5 Management of patients with painful bladder syndrome

available for treatment indicate that no one treatment is clearly superior to any other, and trials of therapies are essentially empirical. There is a dearth of large-scale controlled trials in this area.

REFERENCES

1. George NJR. Preface. In George NJR, Gosling JA, eds: Sensory Disorders of the Bladder and Urethra. Berlin: Springer-Verlag, 1986: vii.

2. Abrams PH, Cardozo L, Fall M, et al. The standardisation of terminology of lower urinary tract function: report from the Standardization Sub-committee of the International Continence Society. Neurourol Neurodyn 2002; 21: 167–78.

3. Skene AJC. Diseases of the Bladder and Urethra in Women. New York: William Wood, 1887.

4.   Hunner GL. A rare type of bladder ulcer in women: report of cases. Boston Med Surg J 1915; 172: 660–4.

5.   Gillenwater JY, Wein AJ. Summary of the National Institute of Arthritis, Diabetes, Digestive and Kidney Diseases Workshop on Interstitial Cystitis, National Institutes of Health, Bethesda, Maryland, August 28–29, 1987. J Urol 1988; 140: 203–6.

6.   Wein A, Hanno PM, Gillenwater JY. Interstitial cystitis: an introduction to the problem. In Hanno PM, Staskin DR, Krane RJ, Wein AJ, eds. Interstitial Cystitis. London: Springer-Verlag, 1990: 3–15.

7.   Oravisto KJ. Epidemiology of interstitial cystitis. Ann Chir Gynaecol Fenn 1975; 64: 75–7.

8.   Bade JJ, Rijcken B. Interstitial cystitis in The Netherlands: prevalence, diagnostic criteria and therapeutic preferences. J Urol 1995; 154: 2035–7.

9.   Curhan GC, Speizer FE. Epidemiology of interstitial cystitis: a population based study. J Urol 1999; 161: 549–52.

10.   Parsons CL, Tatsis V. Prevalence of interstitial cystitis in young women. Urology 2004; 64: 866–70.

11.   Koziol JA. Epidemiology of interstitial cystitis. Urol Clin North Am 1994; 21: 7–20.

12.   Clauw J, Schmidt M, Radulovic D, et al. The relationship between fibromyalgia and interstitial cystitis. J Psychiatr Res 1997; 31: 125–31.

13.   Alagiri M, Chottiner S, Ratner V, et al. Interstitial cystitis: unexplained associations with other chronic disease and pain syndromes. Urology 1997; 49 (5A Suppl): 52–7.

14.   McCormack WM. Two urogenital sinus syndromes, interstitial cystitis and focal vulvitis. J Reprod Med 1990; 35: 873–6.

15.   Sant GR, Theoharides TC. Interstitial cystitis and bladder mastocytosis in a woman with chronic urticaria. Scand J Urol Nephrol 1997; 31: 497–500.

16.   Van de Merwe J, Kamerling R, Arendsen E, et al. Sjogren's syndrome in patients with interstitial cystitis. J Rheumatol 1993; 20: 962–6.

17.   Held PJ. Epidemiology of interstitial cystitis: 2. In Hanno PM, Staskin DR, Krane RJ, Wein AJ, eds. Interstitial Cystitis. London: Springer-Verlag, 1990; 29–48.

18.   Propert KJ, Schaeffer AJ, Bensinger CM, et al. A prospective study of interstitial cystitis: results of longitudinal follow-up of the interstitial cystitis data base cohort. The Interstitial Cystitis Data Base Study Group. J Urol 2000; 163: 1434–9.

19. Buffington CA, Sokolov AG. Idiopathic cystitis in cats: an animal model for interstitial cystitis. In Sant GR, ed. Interstitial Cystitis. Philadelphia: Lippincott-Raven, 1997: 25–32.

20. Houpt KA. House soiling: treatment of a common feline problem. Vet Med 1991; 86: 1000–6.

21. Press SM, Moldwin R. Decreased expression of GP-51 glycosaminoglycans in cats afflicted with feline interstitial cystitis. J Urol 1995; 153: 288A.

22. Parsons CL, Stauffer C, Schmidt JD. Bladder surface glycosaminoglycans: an efficient mechanism of environmental adaptation. Science 1980; 208: 605–7.

23. Parsons CL, Boychuk D, Jones S. Bladder surface glycosaminoglycans: an epithelial permeability barrier. J Urol 1990; 143: 139–42.

24. Parsons CL, Lilly JD, Stein PC. Epithelial dysfunction in nonbacterial cystitis (interstitial cystitis). J Urol 1991; 145: 732–5.

25. Parsons LC. Prostatitis, interstitial cystitis, chronic pelvic pain and urethral syndrome share a common pathophysiology: lower urinary dysfunctional epithelium and potassium recycling. Urology 2003; 62: 976–82.

26. Yilmaz U, Liu YW, Rothman I, et al. Intravesical potassium chloride sensitivity test in men with chronic pelvic pain syndrome. J Urol 2004; 172: 548–50.

27. Hofmeister MA, He F, Ratliff TL, et al. Mast cells and nerve fibers in interstitial cystitis (IC): an algorithm for histologic diagnosis via quantitative image analysis and morphometry (QIAM). Urology 1997; 49 (5A Suppl): 41–7.

28. Larsen S, Thompson SA, Hald T, et al. Mast cells in interstitial cystitis. Br J Urol 1982; 54: 283–6.

29. Smith BH, Dehner LP. Chronic ulcerating interstitial cystitis (Hunner's ulcer). A study of 28 cases. Arch Pathol 1972; 93: 76–81.

30. Theoharides TC, Sant GR, el-Mansoury M, et al. Activation of bladder mast cells in interstitial cystitis: a light and electron microscopic study. J Urol 1995; 153: 629–36.

31. Saban R, Keith IM. Neuropeptide-mast cell interaction in interstitial cystitis. In Sant GR, ed. Interstitial Cystitis. Philadelphia: Lippincott-Raven, 1997: 53–66.

32. Filippou AS, Grant GS, Theoharides TC. Increased expression of intercellular adhesion molecule 1 in relation to mast cells in the bladder of interstitial cystitis patients. Int J Immunopathol Pharmacol 1999; 12: 49–53.

33. Elbadawi A, Light JK. Distinctive ultrastructural pathology of non ulcerative interstitial cystitis: new observations and their potential significance in pathogenesis. Urol Int 1996; 56: 137–62.

34. Lundberg T, Liedberg H, Nordling L, et al. Interstitial cystitis correlation with nerve fibers, mast cells and histamine. Br J Urol 1993; 71: 427–9.

35. Oravisto KJ. Interstitial cystitis as an autoimmune disease. Eur Urol 1980; 6: 10–13.

36. Theoharides TC, Pang X, Letourneau R, Sant GR. Interstitial cystitis: a neuro-immunoendocrine disorder. Ann NY Acad Sci 1998; 84: 619–34.

37. Warren JW, Horne LM. Pilot study of sequential oral antibiotics for the treatment of interstitial cystitis. J Urol 2000; 163: 1685–8.

38. Hampson SJ, Christmas TJ, Moss MT. Search for mycobacteria in interstitial cystitis using mycobacteria-specific DNA probes with single amplification by polymerase chain reaction. Br J Urol 1993, 72: 303–6.

39. Haarala M, Jalava J. Absence of bacterial DNA in the bladder of patients with interstitial cystitis. J Urol 1996; 156: 1843–5.

40. Hukkanen V, Haarala M, Nurmi M, et al. Viruses and interstitial cystitis: adenovirus genomes cannot be demonstrated in urinary bladder biopsies. Urol Res 1996; 24: 235–8.

41. Keay S, Warren JW. A hypothesis for the etiology of interstitial cystitis based upon inhibition of bladder epithelial repair. Med Hypotheses 1998; 51: 79–83.

42. Burkhard FC, Blick N, Hochreiter WW, Studer UE. Urinary urgency and frequency, and chronic and/or pelvic pain in females. Can doxycycline help? J Urol 2004; 172: 232–5.

43. Wyndaele JJ, De Wachter S. The basics behind bladder pain: a review of data on lower urinary tract sensations. Int J Urol 2003; (10 Suppl): 549–55.

44. Bourque JP. Surgical management of the painful bladder. J Urol 1951; 65: 25–34.

45. Nordling J. Pelvic pain and interstitial cystitis: therapeutic strategies, results and limitations. EAU update series 2 2004: 179–86.

46. O'Leary MP, Sant GR. The interstitial cystitis symptom index and problem index. Urology 1997; 49 (5a Suppl): 58–63.

47. Driscoll A, Teichmann JM. How do patients with interstitial cystitis present? J Urol 2001; 166: 2118–20.

48.   Messing EM. The diagnosis of interstitial cystitis. Urology 1987; 29 (4 Suppl): 4–7.

49.   Awad SA, MacDiarmid S, Gajewski JB, Gupta R. Idiopathic reduced bladder storage versus interstitial cystitis. J Urol 1992; 148: 1409–12.

50.   Messing E, Pauk D, Schaeffer A, et al. Associations among cystoscopic findings and symptoms and physical examination findings in women enrolled in the Interstitial Cystitis Data Base (ICDB) Study. Urology 1997; 49 (5A Suppl): 81–5.

51.   Waxman JA, Sulak PJ, Kuehl TJ. Cystoscopic findings consistent with interstitial cystitis in normal women undergoing tubal ligation. J Urol 1998; 160: 663–7.

52.   MacDermott JP, Charpied GC, Tesluk H, Stone AR. Can histological assessment predict outcome of interstitial cystitis? Br J Urol 1991; 67: 44–7.

53.   Nordling J, Anderson JB, Mortenson S, et al., and the Copenhagen IC study group. Clinical outcomes in patients with interstitial cystitis, relative to detrusor myopathy. Presented at Research Insights into Interstitial Cystitis – A Basic and Clinical Science Symposium, Washington, DC, October–November 2003, ICA–NIDDK.

54.   Christmas TJ, Smith GL, Rode J. Detrusor myopathy: an accurate predictor of bladder hypocompliance and contracture in interstitial cystitis. Br J Urol 1996; 78: 862–5.

55.   Nigro DA, Wein AJ, Foy M, et al. Associations among cystoscopic and urodynamic findings for women enrolled in the Interstitial Cystitis Data Base Study. Urology 1997; 49 (5A Suppl): 86–92.

56.   Portenoy RK, Dole V, Joseph H, et al. Pain management and chemical dependency. JAMA 1997; 278: 592–3.

57.   Van Ophoven A, Pokupic S, Heinecke A, Hertle L. A prospective randomized, placebo controlled, double-blind study of amitriptyline for treatment of interstitial cystitis. J Urol 2004; 172: 533–6.

58.   Chancellor MB, Yoshimura N. Treatment of interstitial cystitis. Urology 2004; 63 (3 Suppl 1): 85–92.

59.   Parsons CL, Housley T, Schmidt JD, et al. Treatment of interstitial cystitis with intravesical heparin. Br J Urol 1994; 73: 504–7.

60.   Lose G, Jesperson J, Fransden B, et al. Subcutaneous heparin in the treatment of interstitial cystitis. Scand J Urol Nephrol 1985; 19: 27–9.

61.   Porru D, Campus G, Tudino D, et al. Results of treatment of refractory interstitial cystitis with intrvesical hyaluronic acid. Urol Int 1997; 59: 26–9.

62.   Morales A, Emerson L, Nickel JC, Lundie M. Intravesical hyaluronic acid in the treatment of refractory interstitial cystitis. J Urol 1996; 156: 45–8.

63.   Barrington JW, Stephenson TP. Pentosanpolysulphate for interstitial cystitis. Int Urogynecol J Pelvic Floor Dysfunct 1997; 8: 293–5.

64.   Fritjofsson A, Fall M, Juhlin R, et al. Treatment of ulcer and no ulcer interstitial cystitis with sodium pentosanpolysulfate: a multicenter trial. J Urol 1987; 138: 508–12.

65.   Holm-bentzen M, Jacobsen F, Nerstrom B, et al. A prospective double-blind clinically controlled multicenter trial of sodium pentosanpolysulfate in the treatment of interstitial cystitis and related painful bladder disease. J Urol 1987; 138: 503–7.

66.   Parsons CL, Benson G, Childs SJ, et al. A quantitatively controlled method to study prospectively interstitial cystitis and demonstrate the efficacy of pentosanpolysulfate. J Urol 1993; 150: 845–8.

67.   Nickel J, Barkin J, Forrest J, et al. Randomized double blind, dose ranging study of PPS for IC. J Urol 2001; 165 (5 Suppl): 67A.

68.   Jepsen JV, Sall M, Rhodes PR, et al. Long-term experience with pentosanpolysulfate in interstitial cystitis. Urology 1998; 51: 381–7.

69.   Theoharides TC, Sant GR. Hydroxyzine therapy for interstitial cystitis. Urology 1997; 49 (5A Suppl): 108–10.

70.   Minogiannis P, El-Mansoury M, Betances JA, et al. Hydroxyzine inhibits neurogenic bladder mast cell activation. Int J Immunopharmacol 1998; 20: 553–63.

71.   Lewi HJ. Cimetidine in the treatment of interstitial cystitis. Br J Urol 1996; 77 (Suppl 1): 28.

72.   Bouchelouche K, Nordling J, Hald T, Bouchelouche P. The cysteinyl leukotriene D4 receptor antagonist montelukast for the treatment of interstitial cystitis. J Urol 2001; 166: 1734–7.

73.   Foster HE, Smith S, Wheeler M, Weiis RM. Nitric acid and interstitial cystitis. Adv Urol 1997; 10: 1–25.

74.   Ueda T, Tamaki M, Ogawa O, et al. Improvement of interstitial cystitis symptoms and problems that developed during treatment with oral IPD-1151T. J Urol 2000; 164: 1917–20.

75. Moran PA, Dwyer PL, Carey MP, et al. Oral methotrexate in the management of refractory interstitial cystitis. Aust NZ J Obstet Gynaecol 1999; 39: 468–71.

76. Sairanen J, Forsell T, Ruutu M. Long-term outcome of patients with interstitial cystitis treated with low dose cyclosporine A. J Urol 2004; 171: 2138–41.

77. Moldwin RM, Sant GR. Interstitial cystitis: a pathophysiology and treatment update. Clin Obstet Gynecol 2002; 45: 259–72.

78. Sant GR, LaRock DR. Standard intravesical therapies for interstitial cystitis. Urol Clin North Am 1994; 21: 73–83.

79. Oyama IA, Rejba A, Lukban JC, et al. Modified Thiele massage as therapeutic intervention for female patients with interstitial cystitis and high-tone pelvic floor dysfunction. Urology 2004; 64: 862–5.

80. Ripoll E, Mahowald D. Hatha Yoga therapy management of urologic disorders. World J Urol 2002; 20: 306–9.

81. Lynch DF. Empowering the patient: hypnosis in the management of cancer, surgical disease and chronic pain. Am J Clin Hypn 1999; 42: 122–30.

82. Geirsson G, Wang YH, Lindstrom S, Fall M. Traditional acupuncture and electrical stimulation of the posterior tibial nerve. A trial in chronic interstitial cystitis. Scand J Urol Nephrol 1993; 27: 67–70.

83. Peters KM, Carey JM, Konstandt DB. Sacral neuromodulation for the treatment of refractory interstitial cystitis: outcomes based on technique. Int Urogynecol J Pelvic Floor Dysfunct 2003; 14: 223–8.

84. Whitmore KE, Payne CK, Diokno AC, Lukban JC. Sacral neuromodulation in patients with interstitial cystitis: a multicenter clinical trial. Int Urogynecol J Pelvic Floor Dysfunct 2003; 14: 305–8.

85. Peters KM, Diokno AC, Steinert BW, Gonzalez JA. The efficacy of intravesical bacillus Calmette-Guerin in the treatment of interstitial cystitis: long-term follow-up. J Urol 1998; 159: 1483–6.

86. Rauscher M. Anti-IgE therapy curbs interstitial cystitis symptoms: Case Report. Presented at the American Academy of Allergy, Asthma and Immunology 61st Annual Meeting, 2004.

87. Glemain P, Riviere C, Lenormand L, et al. Prolonged hydrodistension of the bladder for symptomatic treatment of interstitial cystitis: efficacy at 6 months and 1 year. Eur Urol 2002; 41: 79–84.

88. Dunn M, Ramsden PD, Roberts JB, et al. Interstitial cystitis, treated by prolonged bladder distension. Br J Urol 1977; 49: 641–5.

89. McCahy PJ, Styles RA. Prolonged bladder distension: experience of the treatment of detrusor overactivity and interstitial cystitis. Eur Urol 1995; 28: 325–7.

90. Van Ophoven A, Oberpenning F, Hertle L. Long-term results of trigone-preserving orthotopic substitution enterocystoplasty for interstitial cystitis. J Urol 2002; 167 (2 Pt 1): 603–7.

91. Linn JF, Hohenfellner M, Roth S, et al. Treatment of interstitial cystitis: comparison of subtrigonal and supratrigonal cystectomy combined with orthotopic bladder substitution. J Urol 1998; 159: 774–8.

92. Lazzeri M, Beneforti P, Benaim G, et al. Intravesical capsaicin for treatment of severe bladder pain: a randomized placebo controlled study. J Urol 1996; 156: 947–52.

93. Lazzeri M, Beneforti P, Spinelli M, et al. Intravesical resiniferatoxin for treatment of hypersensitive disorder: a randomized placebo controlled study. J Urol 2000; 164: 676–9.

94. Smith CP, Radziszewski P, Borkowski A, et al. Botulinum toxin has an antinociceptive effects in treating interstitial cystitis. Urology 2004; 64: 871–5.

8 | Colorectal causes of chronic pelvic pain

Daniel J Fletcher, Andrew J Shorthouse

INTRODUCTION

Chronic pelvic pain is a significant drain on resources, affecting 38 per 1000 of the general population, a prevalence equivalent to asthma or chronic back pain[1]. A high proportion of cases have a poorly understood functional etiology due to multifactorial pathophysiology. Treatment is therefore often difficult and unsuccessful, especially if investigations are negative or their significance uncertain. A multidisciplinary team (MDT) approach to management may result in better outcome[2].

This chapter details colorectal causes of pelvic pain, which can broadly be divided into organic and functional. Organic conditions may be due to inflammatory or neoplastic processes. Examples of the former include inflammatory bowel disease, particularly Crohn's disease, complicated diverticulitis or endometriosis; the latter is discussed in more detail in Chapter 5.

Functional causes of chronic pelvic pain may have associated mechanical components, such as rectocele or rectal intussusception, and there may be difficulty in deciding whether these associations are primary or secondary developments. The syndromes are ill-defined and nomenclature is confused, with a significant overlap of symptoms. They include levator syndrome, proctalgia fugax and obstructed defecation syndrome (ODS). Rectal intussusception and, much less commonly, solitary rectal ulcer syndrome may form part or the entire mechanical component of ODS.

Intensive investigation may fail to identify a cause of chronic pelvic pain (chronic idiopathic rectal pain). Many of these patients have a depressive illness, but it is usually impossible to determine whether this is primary or secondary to chronic pain.

Neurological causes include pudendal neuropathy. The pudendal nerves supply the pelvic floor muscles (levators, puborectalis and external anal sphincter complex). The nerves exit the bony pelvis at the ischial spine, which is a fixed point. Pelvic floor descent may be excessive during delivery, or from chronic straining at stool, and the nerve is stretched, causing neuropathic damage to the pelvic floor muscles. Bowel dysfunction with ODS or fecal incontinence follows, but sensory damage may also result in pelvic pain. Other neurological conditions seen much less frequently by the colorectal surgeon include demyelinating disorders. Referred pain from degenerative spine disease needs to be considered. Another orthopedic condition, which is sometimes difficult to differentiate from levator syndrome or proctalgia fugax, is coccygodynia.

CLINICAL PRESENTATION

A systematic history is essential, and a well-designed proforma is useful for a consistent and comprehensive record of symptoms. Often the diagnosis becomes apparent when symptomatology is collated, even before the patient has been examined or investigated.

Many patients with pelvic pain have disordered defecation, and the symptom complex of straining, obstructed defecation, incomplete evacuation and digitation to assist evacuation is common to most of the functional disorders, and particularly in patients who are found to have a mechanical component such as rectocele or intussusception on sigmoidoproctoscopy and defecating proctography.

Self-digitation may be per rectum, per vaginam or exerting pressure on the perineum to aid defecation. Vaginal digitation is sometimes volunteered by patients as an effective means of emptying a rectocele, and predicts successful outcome from rectocele repair when performed for ODS.

Altered bowel habit, particularly when diarrhea is dominant in conjunction with pelvic pain, suggests an organic cause, such as inflammatory bowel disease, other forms of proctocolitis or neoplasia. The presence of blood, mucus and tenesmus increase this possibility, particularly when the blood is altered or mixed with the stool. Functional conditions, which may also produce diarrhea, blood and mucus, are solitary rectal ulcer syndrome (SRUS) and endometriosis, although the latter will be cyclical with menstruation. Irritable bowel syndrome (IBS) can also be cyclical to some extent. The symptom complex of IBS (Rome criteria)[3] is included as part of our outpatient history proforma. IBS may be associated with pelvic pain. Examination and investigation are usually negative, although solitary rectal ulcer, ODS and rectal intussusception often have an IBS component.

The nature of pain in SRUS is usually described as a hot golf ball or rod in the rectum, from the pelvic floor to the lower abdomen. The same type of pain may be found in association with rectal intussusception. Patients with levator syndrome also describe the feeling of an object in the rectum, which tends to be worse on sitting.

There is usually no problem differentiating anal pain due to chronic fissure *in ano* from the other causes of pelvic pain. Anal fissure pain is sharp, occurs on defecation and generally is located at the anal verge, although proximal radiation no further than pelvic floor level may be found. Fresh bleeding with pain is usual.

Pain from an anorectal abscess tends to be deeper, especially if there is a supralevator extension. Although a purulent discharge from one or multiple external perianal openings is usual, there may be no external signs of a complex fistula *in ano*, and diagnosis rests on digital rectal examination and magnetic resonance imaging (MRI).

Pelvic pain, as distinct from abdominal pain due to inflammatory conditions such as Crohn's disease or diverticulitis, is suggestive of fistulation and abscess formation. Crohn's disease most commonly affects the terminal ileum, and may fistulate from there into any adjacent organ to involve the adnexae, vagina, bladder, sigmoid or rectum, or more deeply into the pelvis to involve the pararectal and paravaginal planes. Perforated diverticulitis with unrecognized pelvic abscess formation may become chronic and fistulate in a similar fashion to Crohn's disease. Pelvic pain in association with dysuria, frequency of micturition and pneumaturia indicate bladder involvement; other symptoms might be diarrhea, or fecal or purulent vaginal discharge. A previous diagnosis of these conditions and patient age will point to the diagnosis. Other inflammatory conditions include appendicitis with pelvic abscess formation, locally perforated colorectal carcinoma (often difficult to differentiate from perforated diverticulitis in the emergency situation) and irradiated bowel after treatment of bladder and cervical cancer, with perforation, abscess and fistulation occurring as long-term complications. Radiation neuritis is an unusual cause of pelvic pain, occurring in approximately 3% of irradiated rectal cancers.

Fecal incontinence is usually found in females with pelvic floor damage and superimposed age changes, due to pudendal neuropathy. An obstetric history should identify predisposing factors to incontinence and ODS, such as parity, delayed second stage and mode of delivery.

Examination might reveal weight loss, malnutrition, anemia or malaise in patients who have chronic pelvic sepsis or malignancy. Evidence of metastatic disease should be sought. A low abdominal mass would be consistent with colo-rectal cancer, diverticulitis or Crohn's disease, in addition to various urological or gynecological causes.

Examination of the perineum and perianal region may reveal evidence of Crohn's disease, e.g. edematous tags, fissures, ulceration and anal stenosis. Perineal descent and lax sphincters indicate pudendal neuropathy. A rectocele may often be missed by the colorectal surgeon unless specifically looked for. Digital rectal examination can detect tender induration from anorectal abscesses associated with fistula *in ano*. Extrarectal tender induration with a mass situated in the pouch of Douglas might be due to diverticulitis, Crohn's disease or a pelvic abscess from, for example, appendicitis. Endometriosis presents as an exquisite-ly tender mass within the rectovaginal septum or elsewhere in the pelvis. Rectal cancers are palpable in the lower two-thirds of the rectum, but are only usually painful as advanced T4 or recurrent lesions fixed to the sacrum or pelvic side wall, and invading the sacral plexus. A presacral mass is usually due to a congenital or developmental cyst, which becomes painful if infected. Neoplasia in this area is rare, but most likely to be chordoma derived from the notochord.

INVESTIGATION

In an outpatient setting, rigid sigmoidoscopy and proctoscopy will reveal evi-dence of proctocolitis, which may be infective, due to inflammatory bowel dis-ease, radiation-induced or SRUS. The latter is associated with intussusception, which can be demonstrated by releasing insufflation pressure and withdrawing the scope while the patient is bearing down. Proctoscopy also demonstrates intussusception in the form of an anterior or circumferential mucosal prolapse, seen in association with ODS and rectocele. Abnormal mucosa should be biopsied.

More proximal pathology, such as colon cancer, diverticulitis, radiation dam-age or Crohn's disease, may be demonstrated by colonoscopy and small bowel meal as necessary. Colonoscopy is more accurate than double-contrast barium enema for assessment of mucosal changes, when multiple biopsies can be taken.

Computerized tomography (CT) assessment is mandatory for suspected pelvic sepsis or an inflammatory mass; abscesses may be amenable to ultrasound or CT-guided percutaneous drainage as a preliminary measure before definitive resection of affected bowel. MRI is essential for evaluation of a pelvic mass caused by, for example, primary and recurrent rectal cancer, a presacral lesion, endometrioma or anorectal abscess.

Dynamic contrast or MRI proctography are important investigations for the assessment of functional conditions causing pelvic pain, and the detection of associated anatomical abnormalities such as rectocele, rectal intussusception, inappropriate contraction of puborectalis and external sphincter on defecation straining. MRI has the advantage of allowing simultaneous dynamic imaging of the other pelvic organs, enterocele and vaginal prolapse in its various forms. Anorectal physiology including pudendal nerve terminal motor latency testing and endoanal ultrasound (EAUS) are useful investigations if there is evidence of pelvic floor dysfunction.

If no organic disease is found, an MRI scan of the lumbar spine may point to a diagnosis of pelvic pain of root origin.

CHRONIC PELVIC PAIN DUE TO ORGANIC CAUSES

Chronic idiopathic anal fissure

Anal pain of variable severity and duration is precipitated by defecation, and associated with fresh rectal bleeding. Anal fissure is usually, but not always, associated with hypertonicity of the internal anal sphincter[4], causing ischemia at capillary level and resulting in superficial ulceration and failure to heal. The exposed internal sphincter forms the base of the fissure. Localized myositis may induce spasm.

The diagnosis is usually straightforward and most fissures can be visualized by parting the anal margin. In a minority of cases, the fissure cannot be seen, and an examination under anesthesia will be required. A fissure that fails to heal, recurs or seems atypical or eccentric may be due to Crohn's or sexually transmitted disease, immunodeficiency or malignancy. The latter is generally a squamous cell carcinoma of the anus, although more rarely lymphoma; other types of malignancy or a tuberculous fissure may occur, particularly in the immunocompromised state.

Treatment of a chronic anal fissure aims to reduce internal anal sphincter tone, with healing in approximately 60% of patients. First-line topical treatments are glyceryl trinitrate (GTN) 0.2% tds and diltiazem 2% tds for 3 months. Poor compliance, tachyphylaxis and side-effects such as headache are reasons for failure. Botulinum toxin (20 U) injected into each side of the sphincter is the best second-line treatment, with over 70% success[5].

Lateral sphincterotomy is reserved for medical treatment failures. A more limited division of the internal sphincter (tailored lateral sphincterotomy) minimizes the soiling risk without compromising healing, with up to 97% success. Caution is required in offering sphincterotomy to multiparous or postpartum patients with persistent or recurrent fissures, as a previous occult obstetric sphincter injury may increase the risk of permanent postoperative fecal incontinence. Anorectal physiology and EAUS are mandatory. An anal advancement flap, which does not compromise the sphincters, or ongoing medical treatment are more appropriate in these patients, although less effective in terms of healing[6]. Forced anal dilatation risks indiscriminate damage to the sphincters and should not be entertained.

Chronic anorectal abscesses and fistula *in ano*

Anorectal (perianal and ischiorectal) abscesses arise from blocked, infected anal glands in the intersphincteric space, and either discharge spontaneously or are surgically drained. Some will persist as fistulae *in ano*.

Pain may be persistent with chronic intersphincteric and supralevator sepsis, or with extension into the depths of the ischiorectal fossa. Horseshoe extensions may be found in the intersphincteric or extrasphincteric planes at any level. Chronic pain results from inadequate drainage. Usually there is evidence of sepsis externally with one or more external openings that discharge continuously or intermittently. High-complex fistulae present less commonly with chronic pelvic pain and no external signs of sepsis; tender induration deep to, and above, the sphincter complex is highly suggestive.

Imaging by MRI, particularly with gadolinium enhancement, provides a 'road map' that correlates well with operative findings. In a recent overview[7], MRI (body coil) correctly identified the primary track in 36–95% of cases, the internal opening in 11–82% and secondary tracks in 65–90%. Endorectal ultrasound gave similar accuracy rates (48–94%, 41–88% and 48–91%, respectively). Hydrogen peroxide enhancement improved EAUS accuracy.

Examination under anesthesia usually identifies the internal opening of a primary intersphincteric or transphincteric track posteriorly at the dentate line. Multiple internal openings suggest Crohn's disease. Adequate drainage will relieve pain, and this is achieved by laying open tracks external to the sphincters and an internal sphincterotomy to lay open the primary intersphincteric track. More complex fistulae may need staged treatment, with preliminary insertion of a loose silastic or prolene seton, which facilitates abscess healing and acts as a marker for future identification of tracks at the time of definitive surgery.

Treatment options depend on the complexity of tracks and level of the internal opening. Simple laying open gives the highest cure rates but increases the risk of permanent fecal soiling. Alternative procedures include insertion of fibrin sealant, anorectal advancement flap or cutting seton[8].

Crohn's disease may also cause fistula *in ano* and anorectal sepsis, usually in the presence of active proctitis. Histopathological examination of excised tissue, colonoscopy with endoluminal biopsy, and other imaging of the gastrointestinal tract may be necessary if Crohn's disease is suspected. A conservative approach to treatment is advisable for Crohn's perianal diseases; sphincter preservation is important because many patients have diarrhea and therefore a greater risk of incontinence. Abscesses are drained, and loose setons inserted into fistula tracts, and subsequently removed before treatment with infliximab. The majority of fistulae resolve with infliximab but relapse is not unusual. Immunosuppressants are given to improve remission.

Colorectal cancer

Colorectal cancer is the second most common cancer in western society with an incidence of 30 000 new cases and 17 000 deaths per annum in the UK, and 20% presenting with metastatic disease. Detection at an early stage results in > 90% 5-year survival for Duke's A tumors after surgical or endoscopic resection. However, most colorectal cancers present late and overall 5-year survival is not much more than 40%[9].

Lower abdominal pain may be an indication of impending obstruction. More commonly, altered bowel habit, tenesmus and rectal bleeding without pain are the presenting symptoms of a left-sided cancer. Right-sided cancers are usually associated with anemia, obstruction or mass. Pain may also indicate the presence of more advanced disease. Colicky pain and distension may reflect an obstructing tumor, whereas more constant, localized pain might be due to local invasion or perforation with abscess formation.

Advanced rectal cancer may be associated with pelvic pain if invasion of the pelvic side wall has occurred, and involvement of the sciatic nerve is not unusual. Pain radiates to the buttock and leg (sciatica). Local invasion and perforation sometimes leads to abscess and fistula formation, with severe pelvic pain. Locally recurrent rectal cancer may also cause chronic progressive pelvic pain by involvement of the sensory pathways in the area. Examination should include abdominal palpation, digital rectal examination, colonoscopy and biopsy of suspicious areas.

Endoluminal ultrasound is accurate for assessment of the extent of bowel wall invasion (T stage), but is less satisfactory for assessment of involved lymph nodes (N stage). The recent development of high-frequency endoluminal ultrasound now facilitates transmural lymph node sampling with improved N staging.

MRI[10] remains the most accurate imaging modality in the pelvis for assessment of circumferential mesorectal resection margins in both primary and locally recurrent disease, and is 95% predictive of curative excision, such that it permits the use of selective preoperative radiotherapy[11]. Advanced primary disease should be assessed additionally by examination under anesthesia when there is doubt on digital examination about tumor fixation. A CT scan of the chest, abdomen and pelvis will exclude most other metastatic disease. In cases of doubt, or negative scans in the presence of a raised carcinoembryonic antigen level and a previous history of colorectal cancer, positron emission tomography is highly accurate[12].

For primary rectal carcinoma, surgical resection gives the only prospect of cure. Preoperative short-course radiotherapy ($5\,Gy \times 5$) in the week preceding surgery has been shown to halve pelvic recurrence[13]. Optimal results and lowest pelvic recurrence are associated with clear circumferential margins. In the Norwegian Rectal Cancer Group study[14], positive margins were associated with 22% local recurrence and 40% distant metastases, compared with only 5% and 12%, respectively, when margins were negative. Lymph node involvement increases the risk of local recurrence and reduces survival, and technique is important for complete resection of the anatomical package containing tumor and lymph nodes. Suboptimal anatomic dissection is an independent prognostic variable affecting both local recurrence and survival[15]. Pelvic recurrence after rectal cancer surgery has varied enormously (3–50%). In a recent overview[16], median local recurrence was 18.5% but there were nine reports in which local recurrence was < 10%, and all total mesorectal excisions (TMEs) fell in the latter group. Median TME local recurrence was 7.1%. This technique was pioneered by Heald et al.[17] and has been adopted by specialist colorectal surgeons internationally. TME is appropriate for lower two-thirds rectal cancers, and mesorectal transection 5 cm distal to the lower tumor margin is reserved for upper third tumors.

Advanced, fixed rectal cancers are treated with long-course chemoradiotherapy, and one-third will achieve significant down-staging to permit a resection. Otherwise, persistent pelvic pain associated with unresectable or recurrent rectal disease may be satisfactorily palliated with chemoradiotherapy. Isolated local recurrence is operable if sacral invasion is limited to the sacrum below S2. Disseminated disease is present in 50% of cases of locally recurrent rectal cancer. Good palliation of primary or recurrent rectal or rectosigmoid obstruction can be achieved with placement of a self-expanding stent[18] or a defunctioning stoma. Multidisciplinary management involving the palliative care team for pain control is essential.

Pelvic pain from chronic pelvic sepsis can occur after an anastomotic dehiscence following anterior resection for cancer, and also other benign conditions such as ileoanal pouch surgery for ulcerative colitis. A defunctioning stoma may be required. Adequate drainage, long-term antibiotics and salvage resection and reconstruction may resolve the problem.

Other primary and secondary benign and malignant pelvic tumors and cysts

Chronic pelvic pain is caused by direct spread to involve adjacent sensory nerves. Usual causes are advanced or recurrent bladder, prostate, ovarian, cervical and uterine cancer. Less commonly, metastatic gastric or breast cancer, or rare bone, muscle and nerve tumors are involved[19]. Extrarectal involvement or direct spread into the rectum or sigmoid colon will require referral to a colorectal surgeon for joint management. Pain character is typically progressive and persistent. Tenesmus, altered bowel habit, fistulation and bleeding result from stenosis or ulceration into the lumen. The primary site is often known but, particularly in the event of uncertainty, tumor markers and biopsy are appropriate. Imaging with contrast, MRI, CT and luminal examination are needed. Endoluminal stents are contraindicated when the lesion involves the lower third of the rectum, and palliation with a stoma is more appropriate. This alone may improve or even abolish pain. A multidisciplinary approach to management is necessary, with involvement of the appropriate MDT, and active management from the palliative care team and oncologist.

Rarely, presacral tumors, for example chordoma, and developmental or congenital cysts (e.g. tail gut, reduplication and dermoid cysts), present with pelvic pain which is poorly localized aching in the lower back, rectum and perineum, with or without bowel and urinary dysfunction. Pain is significantly more common in the presence of malignancy (88 vs. 39%), tends to be postural and is worse on sitting. Sciatica and buttock pain occur in the later stages. Rectal and vaginal examination confirms a presacral fixed mass[20].

A presacral cyst may initially present with sepsis and be mistaken for a high fistula *in ano* or a pelvic abscess that recurs after drainage. Imaging with plain abdominal films, MRI, CT and endoscopy should be followed by formal resection using an abdominal or perineal (postsacral or intersphincteric) approach as appropriate. Mostly, these lesions are sterile, and lined by squamous or columnar epithelium. Chronic sepsis should be avoided wherever possible by awareness of these conditions and the need to excise totally rather than simply aspirate or drain. Dissection after sepsis may be challenging and recurrence is more likely as the lesion may be incompletely excised. Tumors such as chordoma should be referred to a specialist center for evaluation and treatment.

Diverticulitis

Diverticular disease affects up to 50% of the elderly population. It is most commonly found in the left side of the colon and in particular the sigmoid colon. The rectum is rarely affected. Uncomplicated diverticular disease is associated with irregular bowel habit and sometimes colicky lower abdominal pain. Resection generally fails to relieve the pain and conservative treatment is usually appropriate in the absence of documented inflammation (leukocytosis, C-reactive protein and CT scan changes consistent with diverticulitis). It is usually impossible to differentiate pain due to IBS, which is often attributed to diverticular disease.

Diverticulitis causes local peritonism in the lower abdomen, usually in the left iliac fossa, with variable systemic signs of sepsis. Complications include abscess formation, fistulation into adjacent viscera, perforation with peritonitis, hemorrhage and stricture with large bowel obstruction, although the latter is more usually associated with colorectal cancer. Patients may have a delayed presentation after the acute episode, which may have been undiagnosed or mistaken for nonspecific abdominal pain. They may remain systemically unwell due to pelvic sepsis with chronic pelvic pain. Rectal examination often reveals an irregular, tender indurated mass in the pouch of Douglas or even pararectally, due to tracking of sepsis in the depths of the pelvis. CT and/or MRI will delineate the extent of the abscess prior to exploration. There may be involvement of adjacent organs, e.g. associated tubo-ovarian abscess, requiring en-bloc resection. Primary anastomosis may be inappropriate in some of the more severe cases, which then require a Hartmann's procedure.

Otherwise, uncomplicated diverticulitis is treated with intravenous antibiotics with close observation for evidence of spreading peritonitis. A CT scan of the abdomen and pelvis is preferable to an ultrasound examination because it will readily demonstrate pericolic inflammatory change or abscess formation, and it may sway the balance towards resection.

Failure of diverticulitis to settle requires a laparotomy and resection, usually with a primary anastomosis, except in the presence of gross purulent or fecal peritonitis[21], when a Hartmann's procedure is otherwise safer. Gross sepsis or malnutrition from chronic sepsis mandates a resection (if technically possible) and stoma, otherwise the risks of anastomotic dehiscence and its consequences are unacceptably excessive. Resection, if feasible, is preferable to a loop stoma and drainage, the latter being associated with greater morbidity and mortality. In these difficult situations, it may be impossible to differentiate complicated diverticulitis from Crohn's disease or gynecological sepsis. Multidisciplinary management involving the colorectal surgeon, gynecologist and sometimes a urological surgeon is essential.

Sigmoid carcinoma, especially if locally perforated or obstructing, may present in an identical manner to diverticulitis. A contrast or endoscopic luminal examination and CT may also be inconclusive and the two conditions may co-exist. If there is doubt, then a radical resection should be carried out.

Colorectal endometriosis

Endometriosis involves the colon or rectum in 5–10% of cases, increasing to 50% when endometriosis is severe. Colon or rectal involvement frequently causes pelvic and/or rectal pain and should be suspected in the presence of dysmenorrhea, irregular bowel habit, cyclical rectal bleeding or tenesmus[22]. Conversely, endometriosis is an uncommon cause of isolated pelvic pain.

Endometriosis induces a sclerosing reaction, resulting in stenosis of the affected segment of bowel, which will persist even when the endometriosis is no longer active. Therefore, symptoms may remain even when the primary disease has been controlled. The rectum and rectosigmoid are the most commonly involved segments of bowel (88%), in contrast to the sigmoid colon (7%), cecum (3%) and terminal ileum (2%). The proximal colon or appendix are rarely involved[22]. Endometriotic deposits are usually superficial but may occasionally involve the full thickness of the bowel wall, with invasion deep into the muscularis of the rectosigmoid[23].

Examination should include a digital rectal examination and bimanual examination of the pelvis. Palpation of the uterosacral ligaments and posterior fornix may reveal tender irregularity or nodularity. With submucosal involvement, rigid sigmoidoscopy may demonstrate mucosal distortion, hemorrhage or hemosiderin deposition[24]. Colonoscopy is required to exclude colorectal carcinoma, and endometriosis is best visualized at menstruation when bleeding occurs. Biopsies of affected bowel wall may be normal or show non-specific inflammation. CT or MRI of the pelvis will determine the extent of the disease and its relationship to adjacent structures.

Surgical options include cautery or laser vaporization of the endometriosis, localized 'disc excision' of the affected bowel wall for smaller lesions and formal bowel resection (anterior resection) for larger or more involved lesions[22,24].

When an anterior resection is required, excision of the cul-de-sac is necessary in the majority of cases, therefore mandating a low anterior resection. There is a lower rate of recurrence with a synchronous hysterectomy and bilateral oophorectomy[25]. Endometriosis involving the bowel may be discovered incidentally at elective hysterectomy and management decisions may be difficult. A case can be made for synchronous resection of a fibrosed, stenotic lesion involving the colon or small bowel, to exclude malignancy and because more conservative measures are likely to be ineffective. The argument against this approach is the lack of informed consent and, in some cases, the need for formal investigation (including intraluminal examination and biopsy), especially if there is rectal involvement. Approximately half of those undergoing colorectal resection for endometriosis, with preservation of the uterus and at least one ovary and tube, are able to conceive following surgery[22]. Cautery, laser vaporization, disc excision and anterior resection may be amenable to a laparoscopic approach, even for advanced disease[26].

Irritable bowel syndrome

IBS is a functional disorder resulting in a variety of gastrointestinal symptoms. It is thought to arise from a disorder of gastrointestinal smooth muscle perception[27], without demonstrable organic disease.

IBS affects 10–20% of the population. It is more common in the younger age group (< 40 years) and in females (2:1 ratio). Colorectal and ovarian malignancy must be excluded, particularly in older patients.

IBS patients frequently complain of pelvic or rectal pain, but also bloating, altered stool consistency and frequency, abdominal pain relieved by passing flatus or stool, flatulence, passage of mucus per rectum, altered stool passage and a feeling of incomplete evacuation after defecation. Symptoms will generally have been present for many years and are classically exacerbated by stress, alcohol, high caffeine consumption and high dietary fibre. IBS is a major cause of work absenteeism.

Gastrointestinal symptoms have been shown to vary in women with their menstrual cycle[28]. A high proportion of patients seen in a gynecology clinic with pelvic pain have coexistent IBS symptoms. Treatment of this group is generally unsuccessful[29]. Females are more likely to have had a hysterectomy and up to 60% of patients with pelvic pain display IBS symptoms when a laparoscopy is negative[30]. Patients with IBS have lower rectal sensory thresholds (irritable rectum), which may predispose to other functional rectal disorders (described below).

Thresholds for investigation vary. From a colorectal perspective in a tertiary referral centre, the authors' preference is, dependent on age, to request FBC, inflammatory markers, thyroid function, antigliadin and endomysial antibodies (for celiac disease) with duodenal biopsies if equivocal, abdominal and pelvic ultrasound or CT (particularly to exclude ovarian malignancy), imaging and/or endoscopy (to exclude Crohn's disease and colonic malignancy).

Treatment of IBS should involve reassurance and an explanation of the disorder with realistic expectations, reinforced by information leaflets[2]. Difficult cases should be referred to a gastrointestinal physician. The evidence for modifying diet and for fiber supplements is limited. Requesting a patient to keep a diet diary can be useful. Antispasmodics, such as peppermint oil, mebeverine or hyoscine, are usual in the treatment of IBS. Antidepressant therapy, psychotherapy, hypnotherapy and reflexology may have a role to play in specific cases. Opiate analgesics and excessive dietary fiber should be avoided as symptoms can often be exacerbated. Surgery has no role to play.

Inflammatory bowel disease

Ulcerative colitis

Ulcerative colitis (UC) is an inflammatory mucosal disease of the colon and rectum. The rectum and distal colon are most commonly affected. Unlike most cases of Crohn's disease, it is confluent or continuous and confined to the mucosa, except when toxic megacolon develops, and then perforation becomes a significant risk. UC is often characterized by periods of remission and relapse, but may also be severe and acute, or conversely run a chronic non-relapsing course. There is a stronger family association than with Crohn's disease and, recently, genetic loci have been postulated. Enteral flora, diet, disorders of mucus production and disorders of the inflammatory response have all been postulated as causes but the precise etiology of UC remains unknown.

The incidence of UC is about 10 cases per 100 000 of the population per annum, and it is slightly more common in women than men, with a peak incidence in the 2nd and 3rd decades, and a second peak in the 6th or 7th decades. Smoking confers some protection against the disease, in contrast to Crohn's disease.

The usual presentation is relapsing bloody diarrhea. Low abdominal/pelvic pain precedes and is relieved by defecation when disease severity and proximal limit increases. Persistent pain in a non-acute setting raises the possibility of carcinoma. Long standing UC (> 10 years) significantly increases the risk of colorectal cancer.

Extraintestinal UC manifestations, as in Crohn's disease, include sclerosing cholangitis, arthritis, iritis, episcleritis, erythema nodosum and pyoderma gangrenosum. Blood tests may show raised inflammatory markers, anemia and a low albumin level, reflecting inflammation, chronic disease and poor nutritional status (poor intake, chronic diarrhea and protein-losing enteropathy). Simple rigid sigmoidoscopy is likely to show confluent mucosal inflammation. Biopsies should be taken at colonoscopy to differentiate UC from other causes of proctocolitis. Stool cultures will differentiate UC from infective causes of proctocolitis, which may also be associated with chronic pelvic pain. Colonoscopy can determine the extent of the colitis but should not be performed in severe fulminant colitis due to the increased risk of perforation. Serial plain abdominal and erect chest imaging should be carried out in these circumstances.

Management of UC should be multidisciplinary involving the gastroenterologist, surgeon and nurse specialist. A complete review of treatment is beyond the scope of this chapter, but medical treatment is based on anti-inflammatory agents, topical or systemic steroids and immunosuppressants such as cyclosporine, particularly in severe disease refractory to steroids. Indications for surgery are failure of medical treatment, steroid intolerance, failure of growth, malignancy, perforation and, rarely, uncontrolled hemorrhage. Preservation or restoration of bowel continuity is now the preferred surgical option, with proctocolectomy and construction of an ileoanal pouch with preservation of the anal canal and sphincter mechanism. Depending on circumstances, this may be a single or staged procedure, the latter after a preliminary subtotal colectomy and ileostomy for severe fulminant disease. Patients with poor anal sphincters, low rectal cancer, or who elect not to have ileoanal pouch construction from choice, undergo proctocolectomy and permanent ileostomy.

Crohn's disease

The prevalence of Crohn's disease is around five per 100 000 in the UK. Its etiology is unknown but environmental and genetic factors have been identified. The disease occurs in females slightly more commonly, with a peak in the late teens and early adulthood.

Crohn's disease may affect any part of the gastrointestinal tract but, with colonic involvement, unlike UC, there is often rectal sparing. Pain is a common feature and can mark the first presentation of Crohn's disease in the young adult with persistent right-iliac fossa or pelvic pain from terminal ileal disease. As with UC, colonic involvement results in persistent, bloody diarrhea and more-diffuse low abdominal pain relieved by defecation. Small bowel involvement may cause abdominal pain due to small bowel obstruction.

Inflammatory changes are often discontinuous with transmural changes, thickened mesentery and a 'cobblestone' appearance of the mucosa. Deep fissures result in abscess formation with ramifying tracks and fistulation into adjacent structures. The terminal ileum is most commonly involved, and the disease fits consistently into obstructing or fistulating patterns, or both. Proximity of the terminal ileum to the pelvic organs results in pelvic abscess formation and fistulation into the bladder, ureters, vagina, Fallopian tubes, sigmoid and rectum. Abscesses and fistulation may be extensive and result in chronic pelvic pain until abscesses are diagnosed and drained percutaneously or by open surgery, and affected bowel resected. A decision to perform a primary anastomosis in this situation is a matter of judgment for an experienced surgeon, but will depend on nutritional status, the extent of sepsis and immunosuppressant therapy[31]. The authors' preference is for caution, and to err on the side of the occasional unnecessary temporary stoma rather than having an avoidable anastomotic dehiscence and its dire consequences. This scenario is similar to other situations of extensive pelvic sepsis, adhesions, and fistulae caused by diverticulitis, appendicitis, perforated carcinoma or sepsis of gynecological origin, all of which can cause pelvic pain.

Extraintestinal symptoms are less common, compared with UC. Anal fissures (not necessarily painful in Crohn's disease) and fistula *in ano* (generally more complex than fistulae of cryptogenic origin) are associated features, the latter usually in the presence of proctocolitis.

Investigation of Crohn's disease usually reveals elevated inflammatory markers and low hemoglobin and serum albumin levels, reflecting chronic inflammation and poor nutritional status. Small bowel contrast studies and colonoscopy with biopsies are essential. CT should be requested if there is suspicion of an abscess or fistula. MRI is appropriate for investigation of anorectal fistulating disease to provide a 'road map' if surgical exploration is planned, and particularly to exclude abscess formation prior to infliximab treatment. Anal and perianal Crohn's disease is seen in approximately half of all cases; perianal sepsis, deep ulceration, skin tags, anal fissures, strictures and anorectal, anovaginal and rectovaginal fistulae can all be seen and may cause anorectal and pelvic pain.

A description of the detailed management of Crohn's disease is beyond the scope of this chapter but it represents a challenging problem, and should involve a multidisciplinary approach with surgeon, gastroenterologist and nurse specialists.

Medical treatment options are antibiotics (metronidazole and ciprofloxacin), steroids to induce remission, and maintenance treatment with immunosuppressants and anti-inflammatory agents. Surgery is indicated when medical treatment fails, or there is intolerance to medication, growth retardation, malignancy, fistulating disease, obstruction, fulminant or perforating colonic disease, or severe hemorrhage. Bowel preservation is important, limiting resections to diseased areas, employing strictureplasty where appropriate for short strictures, aiming to preserve bowel length and ultimately minimizing the risk of short bowel syndrome in the minority who require multiple resections for recurrence. Abscesses should be drained preoperatively and percutaneously if possible to facilitate safe primary anastomosis, and perioperative nutrition given enterally or parenterally as required. There is now evidence that resection may be deferred or optimized by infliximab, which results in the closure of up to two-thirds of abdominal fistulae, with suppression of active disease, but which tends to result in relapse unless repeated cycles are given or remission is maintained by immunosuppressants[32]. The same is true of fistulating anal disease. Infliximab induces closure of half to two-thirds, but tracks persist on MRI and EAUS. Infliximab is less successful in the treatment of rectovaginal fistula. Active proctitis and sepsis should be controlled to optimize operative treatment by a full- or partial-thickness anorectal advancement flap, or layered closure per vaginam. There is no good evidence that a temporary stoma protects against failure[33].

Diversion proctocolitis

The majority of cases of diversion proctocolitis involve a rectal remnant after Hartmann's procedure, but the entire large bowel may be affected with a defunctioning ileostomy and retained colon and rectum. It is often asymptomatic but can produce pelvic pain, tenesmus and blood or mucus per rectum[34]. Anti-inflammatory medical management can help but the most effective treatment is restoration of intestinal continuity or excision. Concretion of mucus in the defunctioned rectum may also be painful.

Adhesions

Congenital adhesions are uncommon. Secondary adhesions are found far more frequently and result from any surgical procedure requiring entry into the abdominal cavity or from any abdominal or pelvic inflammatory process, such as inflammatory bowel disease, diverticulitis, appendicitis, endometriosis or pelvic inflammatory disease. Truly symptomatic adhesions will cause signs and symptoms suggestive of acute or subacute bowel obstruction with abdominal distension, pain, borborygmi, nausea or vomiting. Most cases settle spontaneously. Otherwise, surgical adhesiolysis will relieve symptoms. However, for non-specific abdominal or pelvic pain, studies have shown that, in general, adhesiolysis is of debatable value[35].

CHRONIC PELVIC PAIN DUE TO FUNCTIONAL CAUSES

Levator syndrome

Levator syndrome usually affects females, who describe painful pressure in the pelvis and a sensation of sitting on an object. Pain radiates to the gluteal region, vagina and perineum, and is more severe on the left side. Disordered defecation is found in 57% of patients. Rectal examination usually reveals evidence of sphincter weakness from pudendal neuropathy and levator sling tenderness[36].

Treatment can be difficult, but benefit has been reported from local heat (hot baths), stool softeners, muscle relaxants, analgesics, antidepressants, biofeedback, levator massage, electrogalvanic stimulation, nerve blocks, local steroid injection, local anesthesia, botulinum toxin and sacral nerve stimulation. Persistent symptoms may require referral to the pain team or psychiatrist[19,37].

Chronic idiopathic perianal and perineal pain (perineal neuralgia)

There is significant overlap in the symptoms of chronic idiopathic perianal and perineal pain and those of levator syndrome; 80% of sufferers are females who describe chronic throbbing and burning anal and perianal pain, localized in 80% of patients to variable points in the pelvis and perineum. Radiation to the pelvis or abdomen occurs in 14% of patients and to the sacrum and thighs in 60%. Sitting aggravates pain but defecation has no effect. As in levator syndrome, patients describe a sensation of sitting on a ball. Relief is obtained by lying down. A history of previous pelvic or perineal surgery is described by 57% of patients, while 37% have sciatica and 23% describe having had a difficult childbirth[38].

Examination is unremarkable and, in contrast to levator syndrome, levator tenderness is absent. Anorectal physiology is generally normal. The underlying cause is uncertain, but it may be due to a radiculopathy associated with sacral nerve root compression or fibrosis. There is no evidence for an underlying psychiatric cause, although unremitting pain may result in secondary psychological morbidity. Pelvic nerve ischaemia and previous myelography have been postulated as causes, but pain is probably neuralgic at the pudendal nerve level or more proximally in the sacral roots[39].

Amitriptyline is appropriate as first-line treatment, and anticonvulsants or local anesthesia with steroid caudal injections may help. Pain usually remains refractory to treatment and a psychiatric referral may be necessary.

Proctalgia fugax

This well-defined condition occurs mainly in young men. It is thought to be due to segmental spasm in the pubococcygeus and usually occurs at night or after defecation, lasting for about 30 minutes. It is often associated with IBS. No abnormal physical signs can be demonstrated. Treatment includes flexing the legs, β-adrenergic agonists, calcium channel blockers, amitriptyline, local anesthetics and local steroid injections. Digital manipulation of the puborectalis or psychotherapy may help[39].

Coccygodynia

Patients are usually middle-aged or elderly females with a history of injury to the coccyx from a fall or childbirth, resulting in degenerative change. Severe anorectal, perineal and coccygeal burning pain is exacerbated by sitting. Pain and tenderness are elicited by manipulation of the coccyx, which may be abnormally mobile.

Non-steroidal anti-inflammatory agents, local anesthetics or neurolytic solutions help most cases, and caudal extradural blocks with added steroids are beneficial. Coccygectomy is controversial[39].

Descending perineum syndrome

This condition is characterized by perineal descent, which causes a bulge of the perineum on straining[40]. The underlying cause is pudendal neuropathy resulting from obstetric damage to the pelvic floor, chronic straining at defecation, both of these factors, or a cauda equina lesion (usually a central disc prolapse). Aching perineal pain is a feature, particularly after defecation or prolonged standing, and is relieved by lying down. Examination reveals weak sphincters and sensory loss, which may predispose to incontinence and prolapse.

Investigation should include anorectal physiology and EAUS. Pudendal nerve terminal motor latency measurements may be useful, and biofeedback and symptomatic treatment may be beneficial. Fecal incontinence should be treated initially with dietary fiber reduction and loperamide. Sacral nerve stimulation should be considered in the event of failure, provided the sphincter ring is intact.

Obstructed defecation syndrome

Rectal pain, straining at defecation, incomplete evacuation, fragmentation of stool and the need to digitate vaginally, rectally or via the perineum characterize ODS. Rectal bleeding is common and results from chronic straining. Straining is probably an important underlying cause of rectal intussusception, often seen in ODS. Intrarectal pressure and volume increase when straining occurs against a closed sphincter. Transverse forces contribute to the development of a rectocele or aggravate a pre-existing one caused by a previous vaginal delivery which has disrupted the rectovaginal septum. Longitudinal forces predispose to pudendal neuropathy and perineal descent, eventually resulting in full-thickness prolapse in a proportion of females.

The mechanical components of ODS are rectocele and intussusception. It is uncertain whether each anatomical and functional abnormality is cause or effect. A rectocele is likely to be primary if onset occurred after delivery, particularly if it was traumatic. On the other hand, if the primary event is constipation, then straining and subsequent childbirth may induce secondary changes, e.g. rectocele, prolapse and weak sphincters from pudendal neuropathy. Even though the primary event may be functional, it is equally possible that a primary mechanical problem exists in some patients (e.g. intussusception). An alternative primary functional defect could be inappropriate puborectalis or external sphincter contraction during defecation straining (anismus). There are also other incidental features, such as enterocele and genital prolapse, which may be seen in ODS on MRI proctography. Dynamic proctography, anorectal physiology, EAUS, transit studies and colonoscopy should be performed prior to any surgical intervention.

Treatment options are initially conservative, with stool softeners, glycerine suppositories, elastic band ligation, biofeedback and retrograde colonic irrigation. Antegrade colonic enemata (ACE) might be considered in severe refractory cases. Operative treatment is not necessarily aimed at correcting the primary underlying cause, which may not be identifiable. Surgical correction of rectocele has been reported to be successful in 80–90% of patients by the vaginal, perineal or transanal route, with relief or improvement in ODS symptoms[17]. Recently, stapled transanal resection rectoexy (STARR procedure) has been described[41], but with variable results[42]. Further confirmation of outcome by other groups using this technique is required.

Solitary rectal ulcer syndrome

SRUS is an uncommon condition, affecting females more than males (3 : 1), with a peak incidence in the third decade. Two forms are recognized: ulcerated and non-ulcerated.

Pathophysiology is poorly understood, but is characterized by disordered defecation associated with a spectrum of underlying phenomena: failure of evacuation (50%), rectal intussusception (50–80%), pelvic floor incoordination (50%), rectal hypersensitivity and hypermotility (100%), and overt rectal prolapse (6–39%)[43]. Any of these factors, alone or in combination, may precipitate tenesmus and the need for repetitive straining. Failure of evacuation, however, is inconsistent and may occur with or without ulceration, and also in non-SRUS patients as anismus. Evacuation failure is thought to be caused by inappropriate contraction of puborectalis and/or the external sphincter on straining to evacuate ('puborectalis paradox') and may be demonstrated by electromyography (EMG) and video-proctography. This is an association but does not prove any cause–effect relationship. Furthermore, it is also seen in 50% of normal subjects, 76% of cases of ODS without SRUS changes and 47% of cases of idiopathic perineal pain with no disordered defecation. Most studies of evacuation failure have been carried out in the left lateral position, which is unphysiological. On the other hand, Womack et al. demonstrated increased external sphincter activity in eight of 11 cases of ulcerated and three of seven cases of non-ulcerated SRUS using seated video-proctography and EMG[44]. High mean rectal voiding pressures were seen in all patients and high transmural pressures were demonstrated across the prolapsing rectal wall, predisposing to ulceration. Prolapse is found to a variable degree in SRUS, but may be absent. Full-thickness rectal prolapse may be the end result of SRUS, at least in some cases.

Ulceration may be due to repetitive trauma from high intrarectal pressures and shearing forces applied to the leading edge of the intussusception during straining. Ischemia may result from inappropriate external anal sphincter rather than puborectalis contraction, although the histological changes of SRUS are inconsistent with ischemia. Digitation is found in 50–70% of patients and is probably a consequence rather than a cause of ulceration from direct trauma. No SRUS is found after anoreceptive intercourse or in paraplegics[45]. High-grade rectal intussusception is significantly associated with an abnormally thickened internal anal sphincter (IAS) found on EAUS. A thickened IAS, therefore, may be a significant mechanical cause of evacuation failure, and therefore may influence the development of SRUS[46].

Clinical presentation of SRUS is well defined, with rectal bleeding, mucus, tenesmus, disordered defecation (excessive, prolonged straining and multiple visits to the lavatory), a sense of incomplete evacuation, digitation (50–70%), fecal incontinence (50%) and IBS symptoms. Rectal pain is found in 20% of patients. Psychological disturbance is common. Weak sphincters, perineal descent and overt rectal prolapse (34%) may be present, best demonstrated by straining down upright on a commode.

Investigation begins with sigmoidoproctoscopy. This typically reveals excessive mucus, mucosal reddening and an anterior, and occasionally circumferential, shallow irregular area of ulceration on the apex of a mid-rectal valve, which intussuscepts when insufflation is released. Biopsy differentiates SRUS from inflammatory bowel disease, radiation change, infections (e.g. amebiasis, schistosomiasis), neoplasms, endometriosis and stercoral ulceration. EAUS can be used to differentiate SRUS from tumor in difficult cases: five discrete intact layers with a diffusely thickened muscularis propria are seen in SRUS. Defecating proctography will demonstrate internal intussusception and inappropriate puborectalis contraction. Anorectal physiology should be performed if surgery is being considered; sphincter weakness (due to pudendal neuropathy from straining) and rectal hypersensitivity/hypermotility are typical. Colonoscopy confirms an otherwise normal colon[47].

Histopathology shows a thickened lamina propria expanded by collagen deposition from fibroblasts and smooth muscle derived from the muscularis mucosae, which orientate at right angles between the glands. Goblet cell depletion and epithelial hyperplasia are present. Colitis cystica profunda is a variant of SRUS caused by mucous gland entrapment in the submucosa resulting in a polypoid intraluminal mass, which can be mistaken for malignancy.

Treatment is difficult and usually conservative, with bulking agents, glycerine suppositories and advice to avoid straining. The aim is to minimize symptoms, as cure is often impossible. Time should be allowed for detailed explanation of the condition to the patient, emphasizing the progressive damage caused by straining. Specialist nurse support is helpful, and biofeedback should be used especially if inappropriate puborectalis or external sphincter activity has been demonstrated on proctography or EAUS, and simple conservative measures have failed. Other simple approaches such as sucralfate enemas, argon plasma coagulation or laser treatment may succeed, but further evidence for their efficacy is required[47].

Recent results of long-term follow-up after biofeedback for SRUS have shown that 31% of patients were asymptomatic, 30% improved and 39% failed at 9 months, but at 36 months only 7% were asymptomatic, 39% maintained some improvement and 54% failed[48].

Consensus is emerging in favor of surgery for failed conservative treatment, but only when internal intussusception or overt prolapse is clearly evident, in the absence of 'puborectalis paradox' (anismus) and with severe intractable symptoms. Rectopexy is the favored approach. The risks, benefits and success rates must be clearly explained, as surgery may also fail, ultimately leading to a stoma in a proportion of patients. Rectopexy successfully corrects prolapse and alters rectal configuration, but both factors appear unrelated to functional outcome. Prolonged preoperative evacuation on proctography predicts a poor result.

Sitzler *et al.* reviewed St Marks' long-term follow-up of surgical treatment for SRUS[47]. Most were treated by rectopexy (49 of 66), of which 22 (43%) failed. Nineteen (86%) of these had further surgery. Four (21%) had low anterior resection and three failed. Eleven (58%) had a stoma and four (21%) had other procedures. Ultimately, 14 of 19 (74%) rectopexy failures were given a stoma. Delorme's procedure (mucosectomy and plication of the prolapse via a perineal approach) was performed in nine patients with success in five (56%). Delorme's procedure should not be attempted for mid-rectal SRUS, but should be reserved for low lesions with accessible prolapsing distal mucosa. Low anterior resection and colopouch appears a logical approach, especially in the event of rectopexy failure, but experience suggests that outcomes are generally unsatisfactory. Four of seven patients in the St Marks series failed and eventually had a stoma. Anteroposterior rectopexy gave better results than standard posterior rectopexy (66% vs. 47% symptom relief), which were maintained at longer follow-up. There was a significant reduction in the median number of visits to the lavatory (eight vs. three) and median time spent there (146 vs. 15 minutes). Only two had severe constipation despite total division of lateral ligaments. There were also significant reductions in bleeding, tenesmus, mucus and incomplete evacuation.

Other procedures, such as postanal repair or local ulcer excision, have no place in SRUS management. Abdominoperineal resection is effective in relieving symptoms, and may be the only option in severe refractory cases. However, more data on low anterior resection in carefully selected SRUS patients would be helpful.

Hemorrhoids

Anal cushions are columns of fibrovascular networks situated in the upper anal canal supplied by branches of the inferior rectal artery and drained by the inferior rectal veins without an intervening capillary network[49]. Intravascular pressure causes expansion within the anal canal, and is limited by the tone of the internal anal sphincter. Surface tension between the expanded cushions provides a leak-proof seal within the anal canal, only interrupted by defecation, when the cushions descend and evert. Hemorrhoids are defined as damaged anal cushions. Their internal architecture is disrupted by engorgement and straining during pregnancy and childbirth, or chronic straining at stool, resulting in prolapse and loss of the seal mechanism, causing seepage, anal soreness and pruritus ani.

Hemorrhoids are not usually painful, although irritation and mild aching may be present in a proportion of cases. Thrombosis of internal hemorrhoids is acutely painful but self-limiting, and characterized by edema of the external hemorrhoidal plexus, leading to formation of tags after the acute episode has settled. Hemorrhoids should not normally be considered as a cause of chronic pelvic pain. They may be incidental findings or secondary phenomena in patients with pelvic floor weakness, which itself may be associated with chronic pelvic pain.

Dysmotility and slow-transit constipation

Mild constipation can usually be managed by increasing fiber and oral fluid intake. Fiber supplements and increasing oral fluid intake are advised. Constipation refractory to simple measures can be helped by bowel stimulants but, if required from a young age or over many years, escalating doses are required to achieve the same effect. Biofeedback, regular enemas or retrograde colonic irrigation may help. For severe, debilitating constipation or large bowel dysmotility, endoscopy or barium enema should be performed to exclude organic disease. Gut transit studies, defecating proctography, EAUS and anorectal physiology (to exclude Hirsprung's disease) should be carried out to differentiate slow-transit constipation from ODS. In a small minority, surgery may need to be considered; 69% of those undergoing surgery for constipation/dysmotility describe pelvic pain[50].

Operative options include an ACE procedure (antegrade colonic enemata), which requires fashioning of an appendicostomy or transverse colonic conduit as an irrigation channel for fluid and laxatives such as bisacodyl. Percutaneous endoscopic placement of the irrigation port via the sigmoid or transverse colon avoids the need for laparoscopic or open surgery. Occasionally, these procedures fail, and a subtotal colectomy with ileorectal anastomosis may be considered, but the anal sphincters must be adequate, as some patients will develop severe diarrhea. Recurrent constipation may also be a problem. A permanent stoma may be the only option remaining to improve quality of life in these unfortunate patients.

Many patients with intractable constipation have psychological problems, and counseling is essential before embarking upon any surgical procedure for the treatment of constipation.

REFERENCES

1. Zondervan K, Barlow DH. Epidemiology of chronic pelvic pain. Bailliere's Best Pract Res Clin Obstet Gynaecol 2000; 14: 403–14.

2. Gupta JK, More S, Clark TJ. Chronic pelvic pain and irritable bowel syndrome. Hosp Med 2003; 64: 275–80.

3. Mearin F, Roset M, Badia X, et al. Splitting irritable bowel syndrome: from original Rome to Rome II criteria. Am J Gastroenterol 2004; 99: 122–30.

4. Farouk R, Duthie GS, MacGregor AB, Bartolo DC. Sustained internal sphincter hypertonia in patients with chronic anal fissure. Dis Colon Rectum 1994; 37: 424–9.

5. Lindsey I, Jones OM, Cunningham C, Mortensen NJ. Chronic anal fissure. Br J Surg 2004; 91: 270–9.

6. Brown SR, Taylor A, Adam IJ, Shorthouse AJ. The management of persistent and recurrent chronic anal fissures. Colorectal Dis 2002; 4: 226–32.

7. Gustafsson UM, Kahvecioglu B, Astrom G, et al. Endoanal ultrasound or magnetic resonance imaging for preoperative assessment of anal fistula: a comparative study. Colorectal Dis 2001; 3: 189–97.

8. Phillips RKS, Lunnis PJ. Anal Fistula. Surgical Evaluation and Management, 1st edn. London: Chapman and Hall, 1996.

9. Wilmink AB. Overview of the epidemiology of colorectal cancer. Dis Colon Rectum 1997; 40: 483–93.

10. Beatrous TE, Choyke PL, Frank JA. Diagnostic evaluation of cancer patients with pelvic pain: comparison of scintigraphy, CT, and MR imaging. AJR Am J Roentgenol 1990; 155: 85–8.

11. Hermanek P, Heald RJ. Pre-operative radiotherapy for rectal carcinoma? Has the case really been made for short course pre-operative radiotherapy if surgical standards for rectal carcinoma are optimal? Colorectal Dis 2004; 6: 10–14.

12. Tutt AN, Plunkett TA, Barrington SF, Leslie MD. The role of positron emission tomography in the management of colorectal cancer. Colorectal Dis 2004; 6: 2–9.

13. Kapiteijn E, Marijnen CA, Nagtegaal ID, et al. Preoperative radiotherapy combined with total mesorectal excision for resectable rectal cancer. N Engl J Med 2001; 345: 638–46.

14. Wibe A, Rendedal PR, Svensson E, et al. Prognostic significance of the circumferential resection margin following total mesorectal excision for rectal cancer. Br J Surg 2002; 89: 327–34.

15. Bokey EL, Ojerskog B, Chapuis PH, et al. Local recurrence after curative excision of the rectum for cancer without adjuvant therapy: role of total anatomical dissection. Br J Surg 1999; 86: 1164–70.

16. McCall JL, Cox MR, Wattchow DA. Analysis of local recurrence rates after surgery alone for rectal cancer. Int J Colorectal Dis 1995; 10: 126–32.

17. Heald RJ, Husband EM, Ryall RD. The mesorectum in rectal cancer surgery – the clue to pelvic recurrence? Br J Surg 1982; 69: 613–16.

18. Khot UP, Lang AW, Murali K, Parker MC. Systematic review of the efficacy and safety of colorectal stents. Br J Surg 2002; 89: 1096–102.

19. Green SE, Oliver GC. Proctalgia fugax, levator syndrome, and pelvic pain. In Beck DE, Wexner SD, eds. Fundamentals of Anorectal Surgery, 2nd edn. London: WB Saunders, 1998: 254–60.

20. Dozois RR, Chiu L. Retrorectal tumors. In Nicholls RJ, Dozois RR, eds. Surgery of the Colon and Rectum, 1st edn. New York: Churchill Livingstone, 1997: 533–46.

21. Hinchey EJ, Schaal PG, Richards GK. Treatment of perforated diverticular disease of the colon. Adv Surg 1978; 12: 85–109.

22. Bailey HR, Ott MT, Hartendorp P. Aggressive surgical management for advanced colorectal endometriosis. Dis Colon Rectum 1994; 37: 747–53.

23.   Graham B, Mazier WP. Diagnosis and management of endometriosis of the colon and rectum. Dis Colon Rectum 1988; 31: 952–6.

24.   Coronado C, Franklin RR, Lotze EC, et al. Surgical treatment of symptomatic colorectal endometriosis. Fertil Steril 1990; 53: 411–16.

25.   Urbach DR, Reedijk M, Richard CS, et al. Bowel resection for intestinal endometriosis. Dis Colon Rectum 1998; 41: 1158–64.

26.   Duepree HJ, Senagore AJ, Delaney CP, et al. Laparoscopic resection of deep pelvic endometriosis with rectosigmoid involvement. J Am Coll Surg 2002; 195: 754–8.

27.   Kellow JE, Eckersley CM, Jones MP. Enhanced perception of physiological intestinal motility in the irritable bowel syndrome. Gastroenterology 1991; 101: 1621–7.

28.   Longstreth GF, Preskill DB, Youkeles L. Irritable bowel syndrome in women having diagnostic laparoscopy or hysterectomy. Relation to gynecologic features and outcome. Dig Dis Sci 1990; 35: 1285–90.

29.   Prior A, Whorwell PJ. Gynaecological consultation in patients with the irritable bowel syndrome. Gut 1989; 30: 996–8.

30.   Hogston P. Irritable bowel syndrome as a cause of chronic pain in women attending a gynaecology clinic. Br Med J (Clin Res Ed) 1987; 294: 934–5.

31.   Scott NA. The compromised Crohn's patient: when to defunction. Colorectal Dis 2000; 3 (Suppl 2): 23–4.

32.   D'Haens G. The impact of anti-TNF (Infliximab or Remicade) on the surgical management of Crohn's disease. Colorectal Dis 2000; 3 (Suppl 2): 7–10.

33.   Penninkx F, Moneghini D, D'Hoore A, et al. Surgical repair of rectovaginal fistula in Crohn's disease: analysis of prognostic factors. Colorectal Dis 2000; 3 (Suppl 2): 36–41.

34.   Glotzer DJ, Glick ME, Goldman H. Proctitis and colitis following diversion of the fecal stream. Gastroenterology 1981; 80: 438–41.

35.   Peters AA, Trimbos-Kemper GC, Admiraal C, et al. A randomized clinical trial on the benefit of adhesiolysis in patients with intraperitoneal adhesions and chronic pelvic pain. Br J Obstet Gynaecol 1992; 99: 59–62.

36.   Ger GC, Wexner SD, Jorge JM, et al. Evaluation and treatment of chronic intractable rectal pain – a frustrating endeavor. Dis Colon Rectum 1993; 36: 139–45.

37. Siegel S, Paszkiewicz E, Kirkpatrick C, et al. Sacral nerve stimulation in patients with chronic intractable pelvic pain. J Urol 2001; 166: 1742–5.

38. Neill ME, Swash M. Chronic perianal pain: an unsolved problem. J R Soc Med 1982; 75: 96–101.

39. Swash M, Foster JMG. Chronic perianal pain syndromes. In Henry MM, Swash M, eds. Coloproctology and the Pelvic Floor, 2nd edn. Oxford: Butterworth-Heinemann, 1992: 449–54.

40. Parks AG, Porter NH, Hardcastle J. The syndrome of the descending perineum. Proc R Soc Med 1966; 59: 477–82.

41. Altomare DF, Rinaldi M, Veglia A, et al. Combined perineal and endorectal repair of rectocele by circular stapler: a novel surgical technique. Dis Colon Rectum 2002; 45: 1549–52.

42. Dodi G, Pietroletti R, Milito G, et al. Bleeding, incontinence, pain and constipation after STARR transanal double stapling rectotomy for obstructed defecation. Tech Coloproctol 2003; 7: 148–53.

43. Sun WM, Read NW, Donnelly TC, et al. A common pathophysiology for full thickness rectal prolapse, anterior mucosal prolapse and solitary rectal ulcer. Br J Surg 1989; 76: 290–5.

44. Womack NR, Williams NS, Holmfield JH, Morrison JF. Pressure and prolapse – the cause of solitary rectal ulceration. Gut 1987; 28: 1228–33.

45. Lubowski D. Solitary rectal ulcer syndrome: pathophysiology and treatment. In Henry MM, Swash M, eds. Coloproctology and the Pelvic Floor, 2nd edn. Oxford: Butterworth-Heinemann, 1992: 305–15.

46. Marshall M, Halligan S, Fotheringham T, et al. Predictive value of internal anal sphincter thickness for diagnosis of rectal intussusception in patients with solitary rectal ulcer syndrome. Br J Surg 2002; 89: 1281–5.

47. Sitzler PJ, Kamm MA, Nicholls RJ, McKee RF. Long-term clinical outcome of surgery for solitary rectal ulcer syndrome. Br J Surg 1998; 85: 1246–50.

48. Malouf AJ, Vaizey CJ, Kamm MA. Results of behavioral treatment (biofeedback) for solitary rectal ulcer syndrome. Dis Colon Rectum 2001; 44: 72–6.

49. Thomson WH. The nature of haemorrhoids. Br J Surg 1975; 62: 542–52.

50. Lahr SJ, Lahr CJ, Srinivasan A, et al. Operative management of severe constipation. Am Surg 1999; 65: 1117–21, discussion 1122–3.

9

Chronic pelvic pain: the pain clinic perspective

Nick Plunkett, Mike Richmond

INTRODUCTION

The aim of this chapter is to allude briefly to the scale of the problem of chronic pelvic pain, to define it in its simplest terms and to discuss emerging pathophysiological mechanisms. There follows a discussion of the clinical assessment of the pain, and of the patient, by relevant stakeholders whose joint remit is the consideration of the pain in all its various manifestations using the biopsychosocial paradigm. Treatment options, for which there is limited hard scientific support, are then explained, and a straightforward model of a multidisciplinary chronic pelvic pain clinic is put forward.

DEFINITIONS

Two definitions must follow, and are interrelated. The first may seem simplistic, but immediately suggests that the assessment of these patients and their pain requires a wider approach. The International Association for the Study of Pain (IASP; the world body that takes responsibility for the propagation of pain medicine) defines pain as 'an unpleasant sensory and emotional experience due to actual or potential tissue damage, or expressed in terms of such damage'[1]. What this means in practice is that the patient's report of pain is valid even if no pathology is demonstrated, and consideration of psychosocial factors can be as important as biomedical factors. The only IASP definition for chronic pelvic pain syndrome is chronic pelvic pain without obvious pathology, which states that in such cases no pathological nidus can be demonstrated[2]. This is unsatisfactory as there may be a pathological cause that cannot be demonstrated, and there may be pathology demonstrated, but the pain may be due to another as yet undiagnosed cause. In addition, painful pathology may be demonstrated, but on completion of treatment may continue to be a significant problem. A working definition, therefore, of chronic pelvic pain needs to be all-encompassing and, simply stated, is pain experienced in the pelvis of an episodic or continuous nature for greater than 6 months.

The definition of chronic pelvic pain is symptom-based rather than disease-based, and will include those with a putative pain causing diagnosis where there is no treatment or what treatment there is does not result in pain resolution, and those for whom current diagnostic techniques cannot identify primary pathology, which could be ascribed as the pain generator. It is therefore imperative that understandable, but unhelpful, feelings of 'failure' either on the part of the clinician (to obtain a diagnosis) or the patient (to get better), with their attendant barriers to good communication, are shelved; what is important is a patient-centered rather than disease-centered approach.

EPIDEMIOLOGY

Recent population surveys in the US have revealed that 15% of women of reproductive age have chronic pelvic pain. Women run a 5% risk of chronic pelvic pain in their lifetime, but this is increased to a 20% lifetime risk in patients who have a history of pelvic inflammatory disease[3]. A total of 15% of women with chronic pelvic pain report sick leave, and almost half report reduced productivity. Given the fact that, in the USA, 10% of outpatient consults in a gynecological clinic are for chronic pelvic pain, and 40% (in the USA) and 50%[4] (in the UK) of laparoscopies are performed for chronic pelvic pain, it is clear that it is associated with massive indirect (work-related) and direct (healthcare) costs. These combined costs were estimated, in 1990 in the US, at two billion dollars annually[5]. The true scale of the problem is incalculable, when one considers the psychological distress to the individual in terms of pain, distress and disability, and the undoubted impact on partners/spouses and the immediate family.

A diagnosis of disease processes that can contribute to chronic pelvic pain is outside the remit of this chapter, but almost invariably it involves laparoscopy to exclude gynecological causes (and fails to confer diagnostic or therapeutic benefit in 50% of patients undergoing the procedure). Other, non-gynecological occult causes of chronic pelvic pain are in the gastrointestinal, urological and musculoskeletal/neurological domains. This last group has received scant attention as a potential cause of chronic pelvic pain, principally because it does not come under the remit of a specific discipline; we have gastroenterologists, urologists, and gynecologists, but not musculoskeletal medicine experts! However, such causes can be easy to diagnose, and we will include them as part of the assessment of these patients in the pain clinic.

MECHANISMS OF PAIN TRANSMISSION

The mechanisms by which pain transmission occurs are shown in Figure 9.1. The evolutionary function of a pain transduction and transmission system is, of course, to act as a warning. It can be seen, however, that this system works rather better for somatic pains than it does for visceral, and for acute pains rather than chronic. Consider, for instance, that a somatic pain of acute onset is very well localized and easily described and draws the medical practitioner to the site of

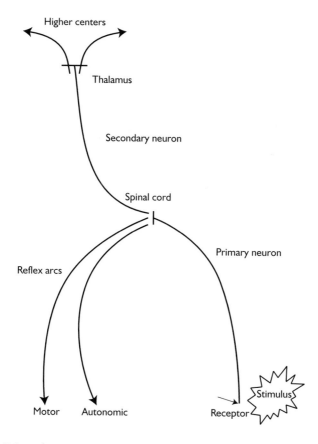

Figure 9.1 Pain pathways

presumed pathology. However, in visceral pain, the pains are felt diffusely, are poorly localized and result in intense motor and autonomic reflexes, which may themselves facilitate the maintenance and propagation of the pain problem. For the patient too the pain is more distressing as it is intuitively less easily understandable, and therefore has a higher fear component, is often accompanied by nausea and is not as amenable to simple intuitive strategies, which can be remarkably helpful in somatic pain, such as rubbing the painful part.

Visceral nociceptors

Chronic pain results from acute pain that is uncontrolled in its intensity and duration. It can be assumed that all acute pains have an organic origin; a tissue process results in mechanical and/or chemical stimulation of nociceptors, which transduce the signal to an electrical signal and transmit it via nerves to the spinal cord for onward transmission and ultimate appreciation of pain. There is not a straightforward relationship between stimulus, 'seriousness' and pain elicited. For instance, severe abdominal pain can be associated with mild conditions such as gas, whereas relatively mild or no pain may be present with severe and life-threatening conditions such as cancer of the colon. On the other hand, innocuous stimuli such as gas or passage of fecal matter can be exquisitely painful when acting on inflamed or otherwise affected tissue, e.g. irritable bowel syndrome. Fairly recent work has demonstrated that the nociceptors in the viscera differ from those in the soma, and are divided into three groups[6]:

(1) High-threshold receptors. These are sensory receptors with a high threshold to natural stimuli, usually mechanical. They encode only within the noxious range of stimulation; that is to say that whenever they are stimulated, pain results.

(2) Intensity-encoding receptors. These receptors have a low threshold to natural stimulation, which is often mechanical (e.g. bolus of food passing through the gut), and their encoding function spans non-noxious to noxious according to the intensity of the stimulation.

(3) Silent nociceptors. It is thought that these nociceptors are concerned with the stimuli that might result from products released in tissue injury and inflammation. Stimulation at the nociceptor then results in a barrage of afferent transmission of increased frequency and intensity synapsing with the second-order neurons at the spinal cord.

Peripheral sensitization

If stimulation is intense enough over a sufficiently prolonged period, changes occur in the periphery, whereby the receptors can be said to be sensitized, or on a 'hair trigger'. This process means that a small quantum of stimulation peripherally results in a much larger quantum of stimulation at spinal cord level. It can be readily appreciated, therefore, that as a result of this sensitization, a peripheral stimulus that is normally painful is perceived as much more painful (i.e. hyperalgesia); in addition, non-painful stimuli generated in the periphery can now be perceived as being painful (i.e. allodynia).

Central sensitization

Changes occur in the central nervous system at dorsal horn and brain level as a result of the peripheral sensitization process. These central nervous system changes can be termed central sensitization. In normal visceral pain processing, peripheral input results in spinal cord reflexes to muscle (usually overlying the organ innervated at the same level), and the autonomic nervous system, which is intimately involved with the regulation of visceral function. These reflexes result in 'guarding' over the area, and alteration in autonomic functioning including blood flow. Enhancement of a peripheral process such as sensitization results in an increase in activity of these reflexes, which can further potentiate long-term pain transmission in the case of the autonomic nervous system, and result in a secondary pain generator if related musculature is continually stimulated. This results in an even greater transmission of pain secondary to the increased excitation of viscerosomatic pathways.

It has been suggested that the N-methyl-D-aspartate (NMDA) receptor, a second-order neuron receptor found in the dorsal horn, may sub-serve the processing of painful stimuli in the normal unsensitized viscera[7]. This is interesting because this receptor assumes a position of primacy in mechanisms of central facilitation of pain of a somatic origin, but is not normally involved in the processing of acute pain of somatic origin. It is known that this receptor, associated with an increase in responsiveness in somatic sensitized pain states, is also implicated in chronic visceral pain. One could theorize, therefore, that the transition in visceral pain from the acute state to the sensitized and chronic state is facilitated by the fact that this key receptor has involvement in both pain states, which may help to explain the high prevalence of chronic visceral pain in the population.

Recent studies have examined the impact of changes at higher centers known to sub-serve the sensory, and affective, components of long-term pain. The thalamus is important as a higher center for pain processing. Studies have shown that microstimulation of this area in patients can evoke visceral pain experiences, such as labor pain, which may have occurred many years prior to the stimulation, and are therefore retained in what can be described as a 'pain memory'. It is possible that continual barrage of noxious input keeps this pain memory alive. In addition, it is possible that visceral pain syndromes have a greater predisposition in evoking activity in an area of the brain called the anterior cingulate cortex, a region of the brain associated with the perception of the affective (emotional) qualities of the pain experience. This area of the brain, which 'lights up' on functional brain imaging techniques such as positron emission tomography (PET), is thought to be unique for visceral stimulation and may be the neurophysiological correlate that helps explain the high incidence of negative emotions in chronic pain sufferers.

Another group of chronic visceral pain sufferers (who had irritable bowel syndrome) were also examined by PET scanning; the part that 'lit up' was the dorsolateral prefrontal cortex, which was activated in anticipation of visceral stimulation. This finding was consistent with a state of hyper-vigilance to visceral events characteristic of irritable bowel syndrome patients, and may also be seen in other visceral pain patients, where they 'scan' their viscera for sensations. Resulting pain can be seen as a self-fulfilling prophecy.

These findings suggest that cortical specialization in higher centers of the brain, namely the sensory-discriminative, affective and cognitive areas of the cortex, could account for the perceptual differences observed between somatic and visceral pain, and provide further evidence that simply dealing with a sensory element in assessment and treatment, without regard to these other facets of the pain experience, might well fail.

INNERVATION OF THE FEMALE PELVIS

It can be seen from Figure 9.2 that innervation of the pelvis is complex, with known pain pathways involving the somatic, sympathetic and parasympathetic entering the spinal cord via a multiplicity of plexi and ganglia, synapsing with second-order neurons in the sacral, lumbar and low thoracic segments of the

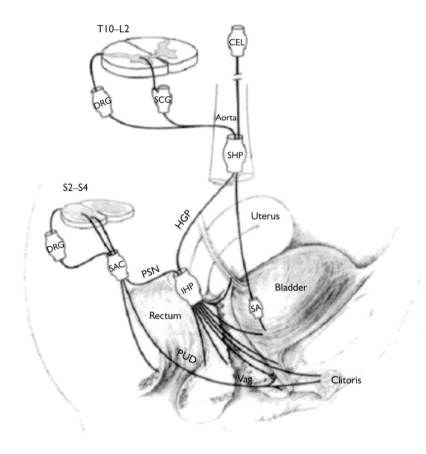

Figure 9.2 Drawing showing some of the innervation of female pelvic cavity and floor. (Anatomic considerations partly derived from animal data.) CEL, celiac plexus; DRG, dorsal root ganglion; HGP, hypogastric plexus; IHP, inferior hypogastric plexus; PSN, pelvic splanchnic nerve; PUD, pudendal nerve; SA, short adrenergic connections; SAC, sacral plexus; SCG, sympathetic chain ganglion; SHP, superior hypogastric plexus

spinal cord. Pelvic innervation follows five pathways, not all of which are illustrated.

(1)   From the inferior hypogastric plexus to the superior hypogastric plexus;

(2)   The pelvic splanchnic nerves that go to the dorsal roots of S2, 3 and 4 and are parasympathetic;

(3)   The sacral splanchnic nerves that pass via the inferior hypogastric plexus to the sympathetic chain;

(4)   The superior rectal plexus;

(5)   The ovarian plexus.

Such complex afferent signaling suggests that temporary neural blockade or permanent nerve section, even where feasible, may not result in relief, especially in the presence of central sensitization changes, as discussed in the section on treatment below.

ASSESSMENT OF THE CHRONIC PELVIC PAIN PATIENT IN THE PAIN CLINIC

Ideally all investigations and treatments should be carried out by all relevant parties prior to referral to the pain clinic. However, where this does not occur prior to referral, other clinicians with an interest in the pelvis, including urologists and gastroenterologists, should be consulted where appropriate on the basis of history and examination. Other organ system involvement may be due in part to the phenomenon of viscero-visceral hyperalgesia, in which hypersensitivity in one viscus can trigger hypersensitivity in another viscus, secondary to shared convergent afferent input at the same spinal cord level[8]. While prior specialist assessments do not relieve the pain clinician from taking a full history and examination, they may reduce the need for the pain clinician to refer for repeat specialist opinions. Such multiple referrals are to be avoided, as they may maintain the patient in a 'seek a diagnosis and get a cure' mindset, which militates against the successful re-conceptualization of pain as a sign of pathology which may be neither diagnosable nor treatable, to pain as the disease.

It is worth mentioning that in suggesting to the patient that they might benefit from a review at the pain clinic, this should be done in a even-handed way without inducing bias; for example, the statement, 'There is nothing we can do to help you any more so we will send you to the pain clinic', suggests failure and hopelessness to the patient. Similarly, the statement, 'Unfortunately we cannot help you, but our colleagues in the pain clinic will cure you', although apparently positive, will of course set the patient up for great disappointment. Clearly, assessment of patients with chronic pelvic pain is no easy matter and requires input from various members of a multidisciplinary team.

History

Many women find it difficult to talk about some of the more intimate elements of a gynecology history. Other barriers to break down are apathy (at yet another interview in a patient who has had a long course of them) and despair (for the same reason). The pain is usually characterized by site, patterns of radiation, periodicity, severity, exacerbating and relieving factors, precipitating factors and associated symptoms. Itemization of medical and surgical treatments, and response to these, can be helpful. Systems review should be directed to gynecological, gastroenterological, urological, neurological and musculoskeletal areas.

Examination

We do not think an internal examination should be carried out without appropriate training in how to interpret findings and, of course, without good reason to believe that it will add to the diagnosis. In addition, internal examination can be intensely physically painful and psychologically distressing. However, many patients come to the clinic expecting an examination, and an external abdominal examination can yield useful information as well as reassuring the patient. The examination should automatically entail body habitus, posture and gait. Obvious signs of distress while moving or being superficially examined, such as grimacing or crying out, are noted, as are behavioral elements to the pain presentation. In addition, this cursory examination can pick up other chronic pains, such as low back pain, and also demonstrate a global reduction in physicality due to inactivity, the reduction of which can become a treatment goal.

The role of the more specific examination is principally to palpate for tenderness and assess congruence in the nature of pain elicited with the patient's normal index pain. Howard[9], in a recent review aimed at a specialist gynecological audience, suggests intensive examination in the supine and lithotomy position, including detailed pelvic examination[9]. Such examination is clearly outside the remit of a pain clinician's expertise. Following an inspection, gentle palpation can reveal two sources of pain, which may not normally be considered prior to referral to the pain clinic. Their diagnosis and treatment are discussed below.

Pain due to a peripheral neuropathy

Pain due to a peripheral neuropathy is of variable intensity, but often exquisite and described as burning and/or shooting, with possible numbness, in a very well-localized area with a pattern of referral that may reflect the function of a peripheral nerve. The etiology of this problem is either nerve entrapment in a surgical incision, or nerve section, either of which can present as a very early complication following either laparoscopic or open procedures. The nerves most often implicated are the genitofemoral, ilioinguinal and iliohypogastric nerves[10].

Genitofemoral neuralgia most often occurs as a result of section or entrapment in a Pfannenstiel incision. It can present early after Cesarean section or hysterectomy as an exquisite, burning, shooting pain felt in the groin or medial thigh, or shooting into the labia majora. The skin over the area may be exquisitely sensitive even to the gentlest touch, and there may be patchy numbness. Palpation may reveal a neuromatous trigger, which replicates the pain. The patient may adopt a hip flexion posture, as extension may pull on the entrapped nerve again resulting in extreme pain. Depending on the site of the entrapment, the whole nerve may be affected, or either the femoral or genital branches, which result in symptoms in the respective areas.

Ilioinguinal neuralgia can follow open or laparoscopic procedures, and is of a similar severity and nature to genitofemoral neuralgia, but is felt as a band roughly over the inguinal area with shooting that tends to occur lateral to medial. Again, a trigger may be found in the site of a scar.

Iliohypogastric neuralgia is felt in a band somewhat superior to the inguinal area and is similar to ilioinguinal neuralgias.

If these pains are identified immediately after surgery, serious consideration should be given to re-exploration, which may reveal a ligature around the nerve. They may also become apparent somewhat later, when fibrosis due to scar formation may involve a nerve. The mainstay of treatment is identification, and often a combination of injection treatment, pharmacotherapy for nerve pain, and physiotherapy.

The injection can either be targeted at peripheral nerve blockade, which is diagnostic and may result in complete, albeit temporary, cessation of pain, or injection of local anesthetic mixed with steroid into the painful trigger. In practice most practitioners use the latter approach, which is simple and straightforward. Sometimes patients require repeat injections (up to three) over a relatively short period of time (e.g. 1 month).

The mainstays of pharmacotherapy for these conditions are the tricyclic anti-depressants, specifically amitriptyline. This should be started at a low dose and built up slowly over time. However, it is most effective at the higher dose range, i.e. more than 50 mg and up to 100 mg, which may result in unacceptable side-effects. An alternative is gabapentin, an atypical anticonvulsant licensed for use as a nerve painkiller; it is no more effective than amitriptyline, but is better tolerated. A month is a minimum timescale for an adequate trial of these or similar drugs, and often several agents are tried in series before benefit is noted.

Pain due to muscular dysfunction

The second system that is not commonly examined is the musculoskeletal system. Muscle dysfunction can occur in one of two ways. Firstly, a viscerosomatic reflex can result in a referred pain, which may become a secondary pain generator, adding to the primary (visceral) pain burden, or it may become the primary source of pain where the original visceral nidus has since become quiescent. Secondly, muscle spasm or hypertonicity, which may or may not be related to visceral pathology, but perhaps to musculoskeletal trauma, pelvic infection or postural problems, can become the primary source of pain.

Referred muscular pain

Referred muscular pain is due to a viscerosomatic reflex. When a pathological process occurs in a viscus, afferent transmission to the dorsal horn of the spinal cord at the appropriate root levels occurs, prior to spinal cord processing and onward transmission to higher centers. Spinal cord functioning can involve an efferent loop via a reflex arc to the autonomic nervous system at the same level, which results in vasodilatation or constriction, and to the musculature innervated at a similar level (Figure 9.1). This can be readily understood in the acute response, whereby, if the thumb is pricked, bicep contraction almost immediately jerks the hand away from the offending pin via a spinal cord reflex. In the chronic case, however, continued visceral afferent input can result in continued discharge to increase segmental muscle tone. These muscles often lie over the viscus, and over time may become painful in their own right. In such a case, it will commonly be reported by the patient that the pain is made worse on movement; this can be detected in the clinic by asking the patient to rise from the supine position without using their arms. Contraction of the abdominal musculature may be painful, and the patient may report that pain of a similar nature and site can be evoked by gently palpating the area. Under certain circumstances, the focal area of muscle tenderness may satisfy the criterion for what is described as a myofascial trigger point (MTP; see below), the presence of which may contribute to myofascial pain syndrome. It has been reported that in a series of patients attending a chronic pain clinic, myofascial pain syndrome, as defined by the presence of trigger points, was discovered in 74% of patients[11]. It is therefore common, and may contribute to the patient's pain problem quite significantly. In some cases, attention to MTPs can obviate a greater part of their symptomatology.

An MTP is a localized area of tenderness within the muscle, characterized by a tender, taut band or pea-like spot within the muscle. Pressure on this, as well as eliciting pain in a more diffuse pattern congruent with the anatomy of the muscle and its immediate anatomical relations, can result in a local twitch within the muscle and/or a jerk from the patient. Some doubt is associated with the precise pathology of the trigger point, however. In addition, the Kappa value (reliability with which different observers can make the diagnosis according to a specific set of diagnostic criteria) is poor. However, very simple treatments can be helpful in reducing local spontaneous and evoked tenderness, and reducing the overall pain burden. These may include stretching exercises of the muscle involved, application of heat or cold, the use of transcutaneous electrical nerve stimulation (TENS), or more invasive procedures such as acupuncture or trigger point injection. The latter involves identification of a trigger point, and insertion of a needle into the trigger point with injection of 1–2 ml of a local anesthetic solution; this, particularly in concert with other maneuvers, such as stretching, can ameliorate symptoms for a time. It is commonly found that repeat injections set at weekly intervals over a few weeks appear to have a cumulative effect; however, it is difficult to determine whether this benefit is a non-specific treatment effect due to attendance at a clinic. It is also possible that treatment of a referred or secondary pain source in the abdominal wall secondary to a viscerosomatic reflex can actually result in a reduction in activity in the putative primary visceral pain generator via a somatovisceral reflex; this is in effect a mirror image to the viscerosomatic, and may occur if activity in symptomatic soma (the muscle) causes autonomically mediated changes in visceral function – a postulated mechanism for acupuncture.

Pelvic muscle hypertonicity

The second etiological mechanism for a muscular element in chronic pelvic pain is due to a primary problem in muscle, which can mimic the pain from viscera. Deep muscle pain within the pelvis may result in symptoms such as dyspareunia, and can be noted by the gynecologist during an internal examination. Muscle spasm has some similarity to painful viscera in that it is deeply felt, sometimes burning in nature, made worse with positional changes and diffuse. The literature on the subject of pelvic muscle spasm as a cause of chronic pelvic pain has some attractive theories, but the evidence, especially for outcomes based on treatments directed on the basis of the mechanism, is scant[12]. In addition, it would require quite a prolonged and painful internal examination by someone with the training and skill to recognize the muscles as a possible source of a problem, and likewise would require an appropriately trained physiotherapist to supervise treatment along relaxation, deep breathing and biofeedback lines. In a recent (1 April 2004) seminar on the subject at a national pain conference, a specialist physiotherapist involved with screening for and physiotherapy treatment of pelvic floor/internal muscle dysfunction in chronic pelvic pain patients, admitted that she had more questions than answers. However, this is often the case in emerging fields.

Musculoskeletal impairments can therefore be seen to occur generally in poor posture and physicality, specifically as part of a muscle referral pattern, and also, perhaps, primary spasm as a potential source of the pelvic pain itself. Assessment and advice by a suitably trained physiotherapist can be beneficial.

PSYCHOLOGICAL ASSESSMENT OF CHRONIC PELVIC PAIN PATIENTS IN THE CLINIC

There should be no more need for advocacy about the appropriateness of psychological assessment of the chronic pelvic pain patient in the clinic. Contemporary pain management thinking over the last 30 years has highlighted its utility. A number of studies have shown the prevalence of pathology in the psychosocial domain, and others have demonstrated in the general chronic pain population, and also in the chronic pelvic pain population, that treatment strategies geared to this pathology result in improved outcomes. The futility of describing the pain as 'physical' or 'psychological' is highlighted by the coexistence of

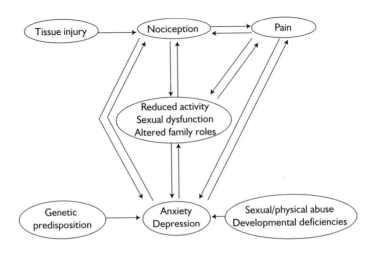

Figure 9.3 A model for psychological assessment of chronic pelvic pain patients

physical pathology, abnormalities of the affective state, poor coping resources on the part of the patient and an adverse psychosocial context. A simple model[13] is shown in Figure 9.3 which integrates some of these diverse elements into a unified whole, demonstrating their interrelationship and providing a handle for assessment and treatment.

Anxiety and affective disorders

There is a strong relationship between depression and chronic pelvic pain. Typically, 20% of patients are found to be depressed on assessment at chronic pelvic pain clinics. One study[14] found depression to be a strong predictor of pain severity and of poor outcome. It is not known with certainty, however, whether depression pre-exists, is induced by or follows the inception of chronic pain. This is because most studies on the subject have been cross-sectional. Certainly a proportion of patients react to their chronic pain and the negative impact it has had on their life by becoming depressed. Similarly, others who are predisposed toward depression may start to manifest this at the evolutionary stage of the chronic pain process. What is clear is that treatment can be effective. This may be in the form of cognitive behavioral therapy or, if there is a presence of vegetative features, with antidepressants. Anxiety is often secondary to a number of other factors and often responds when these factors are identified and specifically treated.

Sexual and physical abuse

Numerous studies have examined lifetime prevalence of sexual and physical abuse in patients with chronic pelvic pain compared to healthy controls or patients with chronic non-pelvic pain. The majority suggest that 20–30% of these patients have suffered sexual abuse, and there appears to be an association between a history of physical abuse and chronic pelvic pain. Abuse history must be sought in such patients. If this abuse occurs in the formative years, it could conceivably alter personality, rendering these patients especially difficult to assess and treat.

Sexual functioning

There is a high incidence of sexual dysfunction and marital discord as a result of the physical and emotional responses to chronic pelvic pain. One study found that over half the women of a large sample suffered marital distress on a validated measure.

Responses of significant others

The chronic pain sufferer communicates to others in their environment with verbal and non-verbal methods. The nature of the response helps to mold future patterns of communication, which may help maintain the patient in their dependent and non-functioning state to the detriment of their rehabilitation. The solicitous spouse in particular can keep the patient in the sick role, the benefits to the patient being that they need not face up to difficult and perhaps unsatisfying areas in their life such as vocational and domestic work, social contact and sexual activity. This is clearly detrimental to the individual's independent functioning. The interpersonal relationship between the patient and their significant other requires assessment to screen for difficulties in sexual functioning, marital discord and unhelpful partner responses, which may be solicitous or non-solicitous. It can be seen, therefore, that the spouse of the pain patient also suffers, and may also unwittingly be a part of the problem. With marital therapy, their limiting effects can be removed, and they can become part of the solution.

Reduced function

The negative impacts of chronic pain in its physical, emotional and cognitive domains can have a devastating impact on function. As mentioned earlier there is an increased risk of absenteeism from the workplace, as well as reduced domestic, recreational and sexual functioning. The key to improving function should be recognition of the factors that inhibit it, with treatment, often of a cognitive behavioral therapy nature, directed towards it. Function can be measured, and improvements in function are highly appropriate treatment goals, and often the best indicators of significant and long-term improvement.

Sleep disturbance

A reduction in the duration and quality of sleep is often noted in patients suffering from chronic pain. Mood disturbance, as well as episodes of pain at night, contribute to a pattern whereby the patient has difficulty in getting to sleep and/or difficulty maintaining sleep; the end result being that they are unrefreshed in the morning, and the burden of their daily pain is that much more difficult to cope with. It is also likely that, following a day of increased pain, the following night's sleep will be more disturbed, leading to a vicious cycle. Improvement in sleep function is a real goal for many patients, and is amenable to non-pharmacological (sleep hygiene via behavioral awareness) and pharmacological (tricyclic antidepressants) treatment[15].

It can be readily appreciated that there are a plethora of problems in the psychosocial domain that may be important in the initiation and maintenance of chronic pain and may be amenable to diagnosis and treatment. Treatment modalities include relaxation, self-hypnosis, cognitive behavioral therapy, treatment of depression and marital therapy.

TREATMENT OPTIONS IN THE CHRONIC PELVIC PAIN CLINIC

It can be readily appreciated that different strands of the patient's pain experience can be at work simultaneously, and can be deconstructed by different individuals working in a team who have a common awareness of the biopsychosocial paradigm of chronic pain. The construction of the team – physical proximity and contemporaneous (or otherwise) involvement of one practitioner with another – will vary, but should include a clinician, who may be a gynecologist or a doctor in pain medicine, a clinical psychologist, a physiotherapist and a nurse with an interest and/or training in this specific area of chronic pelvic pain. The role of the nurse has not been alluded to or discussed in any detail, but he/she can provide an all-important general supportive role for the patient, acting as 'glue' between the other practitioners, and may have a therapeutic role in her own right, such as TENS and acupuncture. These team roles are probably employed to best advantage in a parallel rather than a series fashion. It would therefore be quite appropriate for the patient to be seen initially by the clinician and psychologist, with treatments initiated as indicated, and with physiotherapist assessment if appropriate and a nursing role running as a continuous strand. Any specific treatment effect will be maximized in a concerted, empathic, team approach to an individual's problems. This is certainly facilitated by good communication between the staff members, with construction of a plan with reasonably defined end-points and of a transparent nature to the patient, who is encouraged to see their role as an active participant in the road to recovery.

Multidisciplinary team approach

A meta-analysis[16] has established that the multidisciplinary team approach to assessment and treatment of chronic pain is effective. More specifically, one randomized controlled trial[17] and one controlled cohort study[18] described in the literature attest to the utility of this approach in chronic pelvic pain. The randomized controlled trial treatment was along pain management lines, with the goals of functional restoration and optimization of adaptive and coping skills. In the other study, the patients were entered into a trial of cognitive behavioral therapy with acupuncture and simple medications. When compared with waiting list controls, patients showed a dramatic reduction in reported levels of pain. There were also reductions in anxiety and depression, increased social activity, increased likelihood of returning to work and greatly improved sexual activity. A recent Cochrane report[19] further supports and recommends the multidisciplinary team approach for chronic pelvic pain.

The evidence for other interventions is remarkably sparse, although pharmacotherapy follows general chronic pain management lines.

Specific treatment

Reflex muscle activity in the abdominal wall can be diagnosed as described above, and may be amenable to treatment of internal muscle with acupuncture, TENS and physiotherapy. Identification and treatment of muscle hypertonia is a preserve of the physiotherapist. Nerve entrapment can be diagnosed and treated as described above. Other visceral problems of course require their own specific treatment, if there is any.

Pharmacotherapy

There is no evidence for the use of any particular pain pharmacotherapy in the treatment of chronic pelvic pain, but it is certainly reasonable to give painkillers along World Health Organization (WHO) guidelines. It can be argued that the most appropriate way to give pain medication is on a by-the-clock basis as opposed to a pain contingent basis; this obviates the need for the patient to demonstrate pain behavior to justify the use of medication, and reduces the reinforcement of this behavior. Paracetamol taken regularly may be helpful in some patients. Use of non-steroidals is potentially more contentious, as their long-term use may be associated with gastric, renal, cardiovascular and bleeding side-effects. The use of cyclooxygenase-2 inhibitors may be safer, but the potential for all but gastric side-effects remains. In addition, there is recent and accruing evidence of thrombotic side-effects with this class of drugs, which have resulted in withdrawal in the case of rofecoxib, and a caution highlighted to all other drugs in this class. The use of mild opioids is common, and may be effective in some patients, e.g. dihydrocodeine. However, tolerance is almost invariable with their chronic usage, and the clinician's hand may be forced into giving something stronger.

The strongest of all painkillers are of course the opioids. Their use in chronic non-malignant pain is the subject of much controversy, in terms of appropriateness and effectiveness, especially in the long term. Although they may have been under-utilized in the past, recognition of this has probably resulted in their subsequent over-utilization. Certainly, countries associated with liberalization of opioids for chronic non-malignant pain have reported significant problems in some populations of patients, and even in society as a whole. The concerns are that tolerance, which is a natural consequence in some patients of taking opioids long term, means that there is a drive to prescribe ever-increasing doses. This can expose the individual to multiple problems including, paradoxically, increased pain, increasing desperation due to reliance on a single strand of treatment (which becomes increasingly ineffective in controlling their pain) and the potential for abnormal behavior around their opioid use. Although true addiction (which is characterized by a pathological craving with maladaptive behaviors to gain the drug for its non-therapeutic effects) is considered to be rare, aberrant behavior regarding drug-seeking for genuine unrelieved pain (called pseudo-addiction) is not, and can certainly militate against a successful outcome. These problems are heightened in individuals who have a tendency to substance abuse, including alcohol, recreational drugs and cigarettes. There may be a role in certain patients, especially if they are on maximal doses of mild opioids, to have a trial of an opioid taken on a time-contingent basis. Theoretically, the most appropriate drug for this would be methadone, because of a postulated NMDA receptor antagonist effect in addition to its mu receptor function. However, such a trial should be ring-fenced in terms of duration and intent, and the patient should be able to demonstrate compliance with their regime and an improvement in outcomes.

The WHO guidelines also provide for the use of adjuvants at any point, which, in the context of chronic pelvic pain, really means antidepressants for their anti-neuropathic and/or sleep effects. Amitriptyline is of course the commonest prescribed. Compliance with this treatment is aided by a full explanation of potential side-effects. Even 10 mg can improve sleep but, for a true antineuropathic effect, especially if peripheral neuropathy has been diagnosed, the best evidence suggests that the dose should be increased to the point of tolerance, and may ultimately be in the range of 75–100 mg at night.

Stimulation/modulation

The evidence for the use of acupuncture in chronic pain is not convincing. However, a trial is appropriate in some patients, and short courses of acupuncture, which can be performed by a physiotherapist or nurse specialist, especially if given as part of a multidisciplinary clinic regime, appear to help some chronic visceral pains. The same really applies for the use of a TENS machine, with the advantage that it is cheap and easy to institute a trial. It may be indicated where there is non-specific low back pain, which may result from pain referral or postural change.

Neural blockade

The principles of neural blockade have been applied to chronic pain management for many years. The techniques, which came from anesthetic practice, are applied with much less fervor now, as the results in chronic pain are temporary and partial at best in most instances. The exceptions perhaps are targeted precise injections for the relief of spinal pain. The reasons for the failure of neural block-ade to relieve chronic pain are essentially threefold:

(1) There can be a multiplicity of pain pathways from putatively pain-generating tissues including the possibility of autonomic transmission. Review of the diagram of innervation of the female pelvis confirms this complexity.

(2) Central sensitization. As mentioned earlier, these changes at spinal cord and brain level are not uncommon in chronic pain states, and effectively shift the dose–response curve to the left, i.e. more pain perceived for a given input. These changes occur proximate to the site of peripheral neural block-ade, which would therefore have no effect on centrally sensitized pain.

(3) Adverse psychosocial variables. As mentioned previously these are common concomitants in the chronic pain experience, and supposedly targeted interventional treatment may have little bearing on the pain experience if appropriate assessment suggests the real target lies in the psychosocial domain.

There has been a history of performing caudal epidural blocks for chronic pelvic pain. The results, unfortunately, are usually disappointing for the reasons given above. There then followed a recent vogue for superior hypogastric plexus block-ade. Again, the evidence to support its use is insufficient in chronic non-malignant pain, although it possibly has utility as a neurolytic procedure in malignant pelvic pain. There has been a suggestion that neural blockade be used diagnostically to screen for patients who might be suitable for surgical interrup-tion of pelvic nerve pathways. However, the conclusion from a Cochrane report[20] suggests that there is insufficient evidence to recommend this as treatment; a US observer[21] goes further and recommends that pelvic denervation surgery be abandoned forthwith.

CONCLUSIONS

The pain clinic view of chronic pain is that these patients are best assessed in a manner that reflects the biopsychosocial elements of the pain experience. Applied to chronic pelvic pain, a model for a specific clinic can be proposed. This would require a clinician (either gynecology or pain medicine), a psychologist, a phys-iotherapist and a nurse specialist. It may be argued that this clinic is best placed within a gynecology department, where commonality of purpose, treatment algorithms and a more specialized approach might be most responsive to these patients' needs.

REFERENCES

1. Merskey H. Pain terms: a list with definitions and notes on usage. Pain 1979; 6: 249–52.

2. Merskey H, Bugduk N, eds. Classification of Chronic Pain, 2nd edn. Seattle: IASP Press, 1994: 170–1.

3. Wesselmann U, Czakanski PP. Pelvic pain: a chronic visceral pain syndrome. Curr Pain Headache Rep 2001; 5: 13–19.

4. Campbell F, Collett BJ. Chronic pelvic pain. Br J Anaesth 1994; 73: 571–3.

5. Reiter RC. Chronic pelvic pain. Clin Obstet Gynecol 1990; 33: 117–18.

6. Cervero F. Mechanisms of visceral pain. In Giamberardino M, ed. Pain 2002 – An Updated Review. Seattle: IASP Press, 2002. 403–11.

7. Al-Chaer E, Traub R. Biological basis of visceral pain: recent developments. Pain 2002; 1996: 221–5.

8. Giamberardino M. Urogenital pain and phenomena of viscero-visceral hyperalgesia. In Giamberardino M, ed. Pain 2002 – An Updated Review. Seattle: IASP Press, 2002: 413–22.

9. Howard F. Chronic pelvic pain. Obstet Gynecol 2003; 101: 594–611.

10. Perry C. Peripheral neuropathics and pelvic pain: diagnosis and management. Clin Obstet Gynecol 2003; 46: 789–96.

11. Sharp H. Myofascial pain syndrome of the abdominal wall for the busy clinician. Clin Obstet Gynecol 2003; 46: 783–8.

12. Prendergast S, Weiss J. Screening for musculoskeletal causes of pelvic pain. Clin Obstet Gynecol 2003; 46: 773–82.

13. Steege J, Stout A, Somkuti S. Chronic pelvic pain in women: toward an integrative model. Obstet Gynecol Surv 1993; 48: 95–110.

14. Milburn A, Reiter R, Rhomberg A. Multi-disciplinary approach to chronic pelvic pain. Obstet Gynecol Clin North Am 1993; 20: 643–61.

15. Block B, Wu C. Pain and sleep. Int J Pain Med Pall Care 2001; 1: 56–61.

16. Flor H, Fydrick T, Turk D. Efficacy of multi-disciplinary pain treatment centres: a meta analytic review. Pain 1992; 49: 221–30.

17. Peters AA, van Dorst E, Jellis TB. A randomized clinical trial to compare two different approaches in women with chronic pelvic pain. Obstet Gynecol 1991; 77: 740–4.

18. Kames LD, Rapkin AJ, Naliboff BD, et al. Effectiveness of an interdisciplinary pain management program for the treatment of chronic pelvic pain. Pain 1990; 41: 41–6.

19. Stones RW, Mountfield J. Interventions for treating chronic pelvic pain in women (Cochrane Review). Cochrane Database Syst Rev 2000; (4): CD000387.

20. Proctor L, Farquhar C, Sinclair OJ, Johnson NP. Surgical interruption of pelvic nerve pathways for primary and secondary dysmenorrhoea (Cochrane Review). Cochrane Database Syst Rev 1999; (4): CD001896.

21. Rogers R. Pelvic denervation surgery: what the evidence and anatomy teach us. Clin Obstet Gynecol 2003; 46: 767–72.

10

Pelvic congestion: an appraisal of evidence in the diagnosis and management

Philip W Reginald, Soma Mukherjee

INTRODUCTION

Pelvic congestion is a common cause of chronic pelvic pain and was first described by Gooch[1], who referred to a 'morbid state of the pelvic blood vessels' as evidenced by the apparent fullness. Initial studies by Stearns and Sneedon[2] found evidence of chronic pelvic congestion from the careful histological examination of hysterectomy specimens from women with a long history of chronic pelvic pain, for which no other cause could be found. Pelvic congestion occurs in women of reproductive age[3], and the pain is induced and exacerbated by activities that increase intra-abdominal pressure, leading to congestion, and relieved by lying down[4].

ANATOMICAL EVIDENCE

In this chapter, we will attempt to provide the evidence for the concept of pelvic congestion as a cause of chronic pelvic pain. The network of pelvic veins are thin-walled and unsupported, with relatively weak attachments between the adventitia and the supporting connective tissue and notable lack of valves. These characteristics enable pelvic veins to accommodate progressive increases in the volume of blood during pregnancy, with an estimate that the capacity of pelvic veins increased 60-fold by late pregnancy[5]. These features, however, make them vulnerable in the non-pregnant state to chronic dilatation and stasis, with resultant vascular congestion.

HORMONAL EVIDENCE

As long ago as 1888, Dudley[6] noted the presence of cystic ovaries in women with pelvic varicocele[6]. There is evidence to indicate a 150% increase in venous distensibility during pregnancy[7]. Barwin and McCalden[8] reported an *in vitro* study in which estradiol and progesterone inhibited human venous smooth muscle contraction induced by electric field stimulation. Goodrich and Wood[9] showed that administration of 17β-estradiol in women increased venous distensibility in the calf veins and that such an increase was associated with a decrease in mean linear velocity of venous blood flow. It would appear, therefore, that ovarian hormones are responsible for the dilatation of pelvic veins. Venographic evidence also indicates that ovarian activity is responsible for the dilatation of veins. In a study of transuterine pelvic venography and laparoscopy in 61 women with chronic pelvic pain, ovarian veins were clearly visualized on pelvic venography in 24 women[10,11]. In five women, the diameters of the ovarian veins were found to be identical on both sides. Laparoscopy revealed that neither ovary was 'active'. However, in the remaining 19 women, the ovarian vein was wider on the side of the 'active ovary' containing a developing follicle or a corpus luteum. This observation indicates that ovarian vein dilatation is mediated through the hormone produced by the active ovary; this hormone was considered to be estradiol.

A study by Adams *et al.*[12] showed that in the follicular phase the progressive increase in both uterine area and endometrial thickness correlated with the changes in serum estradiol concentration, indicating that the uterine response was estradiol related. Also, the endometrial thickness appeared to be a more sensitive index of circulating estrogen than the uterine area, particularly in the early to mid-follicular phase of the menstrual cycle. This study provides evidence for the effect of estrogen on target structures, such as the myometrium and endometrium, resulting in enlargement of the uterus and thickening of the endometrium. If myometrium and endometrium are increased in women with pelvic congestion, it could be suggested that the effect of estrogen is similarly responsible for the chronic venous dilatation found in these women. A comparative study showed that women with pelvic congestion have an enlarged uterus and thickened endometrium, and that 56% have cystic ovaries[13] (Table 10.1).

Table 10.1 Measurement of uterine cross-sectional area and thickness of endometrium in women with pelvic congestion and in normal women[13]

	Cross-sectional area of uterus in cm (SD)	*Endometrial thickness in mm (SD)*	*Presence of cystic ovaries*
Pelvic congestion	39.1 (6.1)	11.5 (3.1)	56%
Normal	28.3 (6.2)	7.5 (1.8)	23%

It is, therefore, suggested that the venous dilatation and stasis found in women with pelvic congestion is due either to the effect of excess estrogen on the pelvic veins or to the increased sensitivity of the pelvic veins to estrogen.

PELVIC VENOGRAPHY EVIDENCE

Transuterine pelvic venography in women complaining of pelvic pain has shown that pelvic congestion, defined as dilated pelvic veins and vascular stasis with delayed disappearance of the dye, was the common finding in these women who had no apparent cause for their pelvic pain[3] (Figure 10.1). Using a scoring system for grading the abnormalities on a venogram it was found that venography had a diagnostic sensitivity of 91% and specificity of 89%. Soysal et al.[14] demonstrated that 47 of 148 patients (31%) with chronic pelvic pain had venographic evidence of pelvic congestion, with no other pathology noted at laparoscopy; 93 women (39%) had obvious pelvic pathology with endometriosis as the leading cause. In the same study, 30 asymptomatic women admitted for tubal ligation underwent venography; only one showed evidence of mild pelvic congestion.

Dihydroergotamine has been shown to have a venoconstricting effect on pelvic veins, to increase venous blood flow velocity and to reduce pelvic congestion[15]. Six women with a history of chronic pelvic pain and venographic evidence of pelvic congestion were seen during an acute attack of pelvic pain on two different occasions. The intensity of the pain was recorded on a visual analog scale from 0 to 10, and each woman was then given an intravenous injection of either 10 ml normal saline (placebo) or 1 mg dihydroergotamine diluted in 10 ml saline slowly over a period of 10 min. The choice of injection was randomized and unknown to the patient. Each woman was asked to record her pain intensity on a visual analog scale hourly for the first 4 h and then at 8 h on the 2nd, 3rd, 4th and 5th days after the injection, and to refrain from taking analgesics during this period. Each woman was seen again during the subsequent acute attack of pelvic pain and the same procedure was followed, except that the patients who received dihydroergotamine at the first visit were given placebo at the second visit and vice versa. Pretreatment pain scores in the two attacks did not differ significantly. In order to assess the effect of dihydroergotamine, the difference in pain score following dihydroergotamine and that following placebo was calculated at each timed interval and for each patient. Figure 10.2 shows that at 4 h and 8 h and on days 2 and 4 after the injection, there was significant reduction of pain following

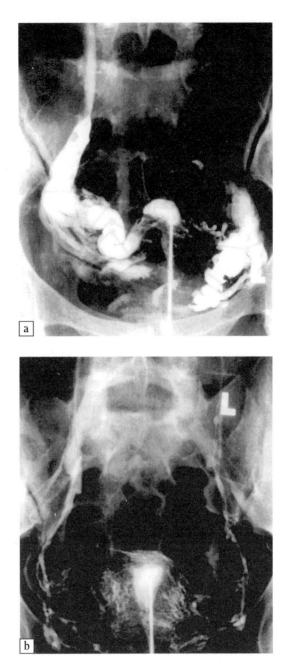

Figure 10.1 (a) Transuterine venogram showing dilated and congested right ovarian plexus of veins. (b) Normal transuterine venogram showing undilated ovarian veins and no evidence of congestion

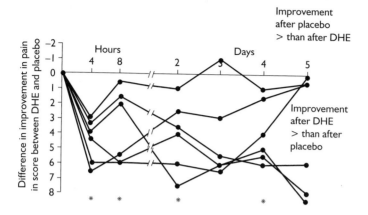

Figure 10.2 Difference between the change in pain scores following dihydroergotamine and placebo in individual cases at 4 h, 8 h, days 2, 3, 4 and 5 after injection. *, statistically significant

the injection of dihydroergotamine, compared with placebo ($B < 0.05$; Wilcoxon signed-rank test). This study demonstrated that in women with venographic evidence of pelvic congestion and no other cause of pelvic pain, administration of dihydroergotamine during an acute attack of pain produced pain relief. This finding provides evidence that pelvic congestion is likely to be responsible for the pain in these patients.

MEDICAL TREATMENT EVIDENCE

As discussed, pelvic congestion is related to ovarian activity, possibly mediated through estradiol. It would follow, therefore, that suppression of ovarian activity should reduce the secretion of estrogen and lead to a return to a normal caliber of pelvic veins with an improvement in blood flow, thereby reducing pelvic congestion and pain. Luciano et al.[16] reported that medroxyprogesterone acetate (MPA) at a dose of 50 mg/day reduces secretion of estrogen to a blood concentration consistent with that found in the early follicular phase of the cycle. A study has also been described in which 22 women with pelvic congestion proven by transuterine pelvic venography were treated with oral MPA 30 mg/day for 6 months[17]. At the end of the treatment period, a pelvic venogram was performed. The findings before and after treatment were compared, as well as pain scores.

Among the 17 women who showed a reduction in venogram score after treatment, the median percentage change in pain score was 75%, compared with a median percentage change of 29% among those women who showed no reduction in venogram score. The improvement in pelvic pain in women who showed a reduction in pelvic congestion was significantly higher than in those women who showed no reduction in pelvic congestion. These results add further evidence to the earlier finding that pelvic congestion is the cause of pain in these women.

In a double-blind randomized controlled trial of treatment with MPA and/or psychotherapy, a statistically significant benefit in terms of a reduction in pain after 4 months of treatment with MPA alone was noted[18]; 6 months after stopping treatment the beneficial effect of MPA alone remained, but was no longer greater than in the placebo group. However, the group treated with MPA and psychotherapy showed the greatest benefit at this time. In a prospective randomized trial, Soysal et al.[14] compared the efficacy of medroxyprogesterone acetate 30 mg/day with goserelin acetate 3.6 mg/month over a period of 6 months. At the end of treatment, both agents produced significant improvements in pelvic pain. However, the effectiveness of goserelin acetate was longer lasting when subjective improvement of pain was assessed at 12 months after treatment.

SURGICAL TREATMENT EVIDENCE

If ovarian activity is the cause of pain due to pelvic congestion, then any form of surgery which diminishes or ablates the functional activity of the ovary will be effective. Beard et al.[19] undertook total abdominal hysterectomy and bilateral oophorectomy in a small group of women who had debilitating pain due to pelvic congestion. The majority of women responded to ovarian suppression previously but the pain recurred, interfering with their quality of life. These women underwent bilateral salpingo-oophorectomy along with hysterectomy after careful counseling. Initial and long-term follow-up of these women has shown a complete resolution of pain with a return to a normal social and sexual life. Although these results are encouraging, they should not be regarded as an indication for primary treatment of pelvic congestion, and it must be pointed out that of the 900 women who had attended the tertiary center at St Mary's Hospital during that period, total abdominal hysterectomy and bilateral salpingo-oophorectomy was undertaken in only 35 of them. The remaining women have been managed successfully by a variety of medical and psychological interventions. Recent reports indicate a role for laparoscopic ligation of pelvic and ovarian varicoceles or embolization of the ovarian veins with interventional radiological techniques[20]. These are interesting areas of progress and studies with long-term follow-up are awaited.

CONCLUSIONS

The diagnosis of pelvic congestion syndrome as a cause of chronic pelvic pain remains controversial. There is growing evidence in the literature that pelvic congestion is a clinical entity occurring in women of reproductive age that disappears after menopause. A diagnosis of this condition could be made by ultrasound[21], at laparoscopy and by transuterine pelvic venography. Ovarian suppression produces relief of pelvic pain and, in a small number of cases, hysterectomy with bilateral oophorectomy may become necessary to provide relief.

REFERENCES

1. Gooch R. On some of the most important diseases peculiar to women. London: New Sydenham Society, 1859: 299–31.

2. Stearns HC, Sneeden VD. Observations on the clinical and pathologic aspects of the pelvic congestion syndrome. Am J Obstet Gynecol 1966; 94: 718–32.

3. Beard RW, Highman JH, Pearce S, Reginald PW. Diagnosis of pelvic varicosities in women with chronic pelvic pain. Lancet 1984; 2: 946–9.

4. Thomas DC, McArdle FJ, Rogers VE, et al. Local blood volume changes in women with pelvic congestion measured by applied potential tomography. Clin Sci 1991; 81: 401–4.

5. Hodgkinson CP. Physiology of the ovarian veins during pregnancy. Obstet Gynecol 1953; 1: 26–37.

6. Dudley A. Varicocoele in the female. What is its influence on the ovary? New York Med J 1888; 48: 174–7.

7. McCausland AM, Hyman G, Winsor T, Trotter AD Jr. Venous distensibility during pregnancy. Am J Obstet Gynecol 1961; 81: 472–8.

8. Barwin BN, McCalden TA. The inhibitory action of oestradiol-17 beta and proges-
    terone on human venous smooth muscle. J Physiol 1972; 227: 41P–42P.

9. Goodrich SM, Wood JE. The effect of estradiol-17 beta on peripheral venous dis-
    tensibility and velocity of venous blood flow. Am J Obstet Gynecol 1966; 96:
    407–12.

10. Reginald PW, Beard RW, Pearce S. Pelvic pain due to pelvic venous congestion. In
    Studd J, ed. Progress in Obstetrics and Gynaecology. Edinburgh: Churchill
    Livingstone, 1989: 275–93.

11. Reginald PW. Investigation of pelvic congestion as a cause for chronic pelvic pain
    in women with no pelvic pathology. MD thesis, London University, 1989.

12. Adams JM, Tan SL, Wheeler MJ, et al. Uterine growth in the follicular phase of
    spontaneous ovulatory cycles and during luteinizing hormone-releasing hor-
    mone-induced cycles in women with normal or polycystic ovaries. Fertil Steril
    1988; 49: 52–5.

13. Adams J, Reginald PW, Franks S, et al. Uterine size and endometrial thickness and
    the significance of cystic ovaries in women with pelvic pain due to congestion. Br
    J Obstet Gynaecol 1990; 97: 583–7.

14. Soysal ME, Soysal S, Vicdan K, Ozer SA. Randomised controlled trial of goserelin
    and medroxyprogesterone acetate in the treatment of pelvic congestion. Hum
    Reprod 2001; 16: 931–9.

15. Reginald PW, Beard RW, Kooner JS, et al. Intravenous dihydroergotamine to
    relieve pelvic congestion with pain in young women. Lancet 1987; 2: 351–3.

16. Luciano AA. Turksey RN, Dlugi AM, Carleo JL. Endocrine consequences of oral
    medroxyprogesterone acetate (MPA) in the treatment of endometriosis. Presented
    at the 68th Annual Meeting of the Endocrine Society, Anaheim, California, 1986;
    abstr 694.

17. Reginald PW, Adams J, Franks S, et al. Medroxyprogesterone acetate in the treat-
    ment of pelvic pain due to venous congestion. Br J Obstet Gynaecol 1989; 96:
    1148–52.

18. Farquhar CM, Rogers V, Franks S, et al. A randomized controlled trial of medrox-
    yprogesterone acetate and psychotherapy for the treatment of pelvic congestion.
    Br J Obstet Gynaecol 1989; 96: 1153–62.

19.   Beard RW, Kennedy RG, Gangar KF, et al. Bilateral oophorectomy and hysterecto-
       my in the treatment of intractable pelvic pain associated with pelvic congestion.
       Br J Obstet Gynaecol 1991; 98: 988–92.

20.   Venbrux AC, Lambert DL. Embolization of the ovarian veins as a treatment for
       patients with chronic pelvic pain caused by pelvic venous incompetence (pelvic
       congestion syndrome). Curr Opin Obstet Gynecol 1999; 11: 395–9.

21.   Giacchetto C, Cotroneo GB, Marincolo F, et al. Ovarian varicocele: ultrasonic and
       phlebographic evaluation. J Clin Ultrasound 1990; 18: 551–5.

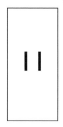

Chronic pelvic pain: the role of psychological factors and implications for care

Pauline Slade

INTRODUCTION

The role of psychological factors in the experience of gynecological difficulties is well established, with high levels of distress being recorded in gynecological out-patients[1,2]. The experience of chronic pelvic pain (pain lasting more than 6 months) in particular has a major negative impact on quality of life. In providing care for women with such difficulties the aims cannot be solely to remove pathology but also to reduce the experience of pain and its adverse impact on life in terms of mood and disability. It is crucial, therefore, to understand not just the causes of pathology but the factors that influence the experience of pain and response to this. This chapter aims to:

(1) Identify why psychological factors are important and illustrate this in a typical process of care;

(2) Provide a brief consideration of the literature on psychological factors influencing both causation and response from a historical and current perspective;

(3) Describe current knowledge about women's own experiences of care for chronic pelvic pain; and

(4) Consider implications for improving care.

THE ROLE OF PSYCHOLOGICAL FACTORS

It is well established that there is no rule of equivalence, i.e. that degree of identifiable pathology does not predict experience of pain. Pain may be absent or minor in the presence of severe pathology and, conversely, severe pain may occur in the apparent absence of any pathology. Understanding pain requires consideration of psychological and social factors that influence both the experience of pain and the degree of consequent disability. We know that there are individual differences in pain thresholds and tolerance of painful stimuli. In addition, other psychological factors, such as current focus of attention, thoughts about the meaning of the pain or its implications, and mood, may all affect pain experience. For example, where people frequently 'catastrophize' – that is, engage in a series of negative thoughts, such as 'this is awful, it's going to go on forever, there's nothing I can do, it's ruining my life' – this leads to intensification of the pain experience and greater distress.

THE TYPICAL PROCESS OF CARE

The typical process of care in women with chronic pelvic pain can be broken down into several discrete stages: experiencing pain; making a decision to consult; attending their general practitioner (GP) once or many times; receiving referral to secondary care; consultation(s) with a gynecologist; investigations; receiving results; treatment (which may or may not have been combined with the investigatory process); and discharge or continuing care. Unfortunately, many women become stuck in a repeating cycle.

It is perhaps helpful to look at how psychological factors may impact at each stage. Women experience pain and after a while consult with their GP. When they consult will be influenced not only by the severity of their pain experience but also its impact on their life and what beliefs they have about the cause of the pain. Beliefs, in turn, will be influenced by both their social situation (who they have around them and their degree of openness with others) and the experiences of others. People may present at their GPs with pain after very different durations of pain experience. Similarly, different GPs may refer to gynecologists after different numbers of consultations. Following referral, a range of physical problems may be implicated and the normal process of care involves an investigatory operation, often a laparoscopy (a procedure involving the insertion of an optical device through a cut in the abdominal wall) through which the internal state of the pelvic organs can be examined.

However, studies suggest that the rate of detected abnormalities ranges from 8 to 88%, with endometriosis (migration of tissue from the lining of the womb) and pelvic adhesions some of the more common findings. In other cases, the pain may be attributed to pelvic congestion, cervical stenosis or to other systems of the body, such as abnormalities of bowel functioning. Women are often discharged from gynecology clinics having been provided with 'reassurance' after a 'negative' laparoscopy (i.e. an investigation of the gynecological structures where no abnormality is found) and no further care is provided.

For many, the pelvic pain becomes chronic (defined as lasting for more than 6 months) and a repeated ineffective cycle of care may be instigated with some women undergoing numerous laparoscopies. McGowan *et al.*, who surveyed GP perspectives, suggest that where there is no clear abnormality women are 'caught in a futile cycle of referral and investigation'[3]. What is very clear is that for many women treatment becomes idiosyncratic and ineffective. In a study of family doctors' perspectives on providing care for psychological aspects of gynecological conditions, dealing with chronic pelvic pain was rated as the most problematic and where they felt they required most assistance[4].

Chronic pelvic pain not only presents challenges for GPs and gynecologists providing care, but it has major long-term impact for the women themselves, in terms of an increased risk of experience of depressive symptoms, difficulty in sexual relationships, reductions in social and leisure activities as well as adverse employment implications.

THE POTENTIAL ROLE OF FEAR OF PAIN IN PREDICTING DISABILITY

One way of understanding such degree of disability has been provided by Vlaeyen and Linton[5]. They suggest that once an individual experiences pain, then fear of recurrence or intensification becomes a major factor. High fear of pain is proposed to lead to both awareness and avoidance with the following patterns:

(1)   Through increased awareness a person becomes hypervigilant for signs of pain onset or identification. As a result, their threshold for noticing bodily changes is reduced and attention, anxiety and tension increase with a concurrent increase in pain experience.

(2)   Through attempting to avoid the pain the person gradually becomes more restricted in their activities as a way of attempting to protect themselves.

(3)   This, in turn, leads to a reduction in potentially pleasurable activities, a reduction in social contact, and decreased enjoyment and achievement.

(4)   This leads to increased attention to the pain or potential of pain and to low mood, with feelings of frustration and anger at the restricted lifestyle and personal costs of the pain.

This pattern has the potential to create a cycle of increasing disability. Certainly, in studies of people with back pain, fear of pain assessed at the first acute episode is the major predictor of disability level at 12 months[6]. Such ideas have clear relevance to chronic pelvic pain and require empirical testing in this context.

PSYCHOLOGICAL FACTORS IN CAUSATION AND RESPONSE

Early research considering psychological aspects of pelvic pain tended to focus upon a search for differential determinants for what was construed as 'psychogenic or functional' pain, as opposed to what was construed as 'organic' pain. The dichotomy that has existed in much of the literature between 'functional' and 'organic' or psychological vs. physiological causation has, in many respects, been unhelpful. The majority of more recent studies have failed to find psychological differences in terms of personality profiles or mood states between women with chronic pelvic pain with and without pathology (for a review see Savidge and Slade[7]). However, there are certainly differences between these groups and non-pain comparison groups in that levels of depressive symptoms are elevated in the former. Hence, current thinking suggests that psychological distress is a response *to* rather than a cause *of* the pain. It must also be noted that identifying pathological causation is an imprecise process, which is limited by current knowledge and techniques. Secondly, the presence of abnormality does not necessarily mean that this is the actual cause. Many women around the age of 40 years, a typical time for consultation about pelvic pain, show signs of endometriosis, which in a chronic pelvic pain patient would be designated as identifiable pathology, but report no pain or are certainly not consulting for chronic pelvic pain.

One particular pathophysiological mechanism suggested linking the psychological and physiological domains is pelvic congestion. This is a condition whereby a woman may develop chronically dilated pelvic veins, which has been hypothesized to occur in response to stress. One group of workers have suggested increased rates of child abuse in women with chronic pelvic pain showing pelvic congestion[8]. This, therefore, remains a possible avenue for consideration. However, definitive venographic studies remain to be completed.

DOES THE APPARENT PRESENCE OR ABSENCE OF PATHOLOGY INFLUENCE OUTCOME?

Interestingly, a study by Richter *et al.* suggests that the presence or absence of pathology has no discernible impact in terms of outcomes in long-term follow-up[9]. Similar conclusions were drawn by Elcombe *et al.*, who randomly allocated 71 women to wait 2 or 10 weeks for laparoscopy[10]. Pain ratings reduced following laparoscopy. However, the main predictors of this reduction were not pain chronicity or degree of pathology but changes in beliefs about the pain and the woman's own evaluation of the seriousness of her condition. Interestingly, those who viewed their condition as more serious showed greater reductions in pain, possibly because they were more accepting of potential chronicity and the need to manage rather than cure. However, the importance of appraisal factors is clearly emphasized.

IS THE EXPERIENCE OF SEXUAL ABUSE A PREDISPOSING FACTOR FOR CHRONIC PELVIC PAIN?

The potential role of sexual abuse in women with chronic pelvic pain has only recently been appreciated. Walker *et al.*, for example, suggested elevated rates of childhood or adult sexual trauma (58%) in chronic pelvic pain patients[11]. In a group of 106 women with chronic pelvic pain without pathology, Reiter *et al.* suggested a rate of 48%, compared with 6% in a pain-free gynecological outpatient control group[12]. However, findings are not totally consistent, with Rapkin *et al.* finding no significant differences in prevalence between chronic pelvic pain groups, other chronic pain groups and a no pain group[13]. The former did, however, show high rates of physical abuse in childhood. Interestingly, a recent study by Raphael *et al.* has taken a prospective view, identifying a large number of childhood victims and following them up as adults to assess their rate of medically explained and unexplained pain complaints[14]. The odds of reporting medically unexplained pain symptoms were not elevated in those who were childhood victims of abuse. However, if one considered retrospective assessments of abuse, then having one or more unexplained pain symptoms was associated with recollections of victimization. This provides one potential mechanism of linkage between recall of sexual abuse and pain. We know that mood affects access to different memories and that there is a mood-congruent effect whereby it is easier to recall memories encoded in the same emotional state. If chronic pain leads to the experience of emotional distress then experiencing pain may facilitate the recall of memories such as sexual abuse, which are likely to be encoded in a similar state.

There are several other mechanisms through which the experience of sexual abuse could influence the risk of chronic pelvic pain. Sexual abuse is linked with both social disadvantage and lower self-esteem in women. Both of these factors increase the probability of more numerous sexual partners and hence the risk of infection and subsequent pain. An additional strand of work by Heim *et al.* has suggested that childhood sexual abuse changes the responsivity of the hypothalamic–pituitary–adrenal axis and increases susceptibility to chronic pelvic pain[15].

A fourth idea also focuses on how women may react to minor experience of pain. Toomy *et al.* suggest that women with chronic pelvic pain who had experienced abuse reported less perceived life control and a more punishing response to the pain and higher levels of global distress, compared with women with chronic pelvic pain and no history of abuse[16]. They concluded that a combination of abuse and chronic pelvic pain is likely to lead to a particularly high somatic preoccupation, and provide a schema in which the likelihood of perceiving sensory input from the pelvis is high, i.e. that there is hypervigilance to discomfort in that area of the body. Early experiences are therefore potentially of relevance in chronic pelvic pain but relationships are likely to be complex and involve a variety of physiological and psychological mechanisms including appraisal and response to pain.

SEXUAL PROBLEMS

A high prevalence of adult sexual dysfunction has been suggested to occur in women with chronic pelvic pain[17]. Several studies have related this to the rates of sexual abuse. However, chronic pelvic pain is associated with depressive symptoms and hence a reduction in libido. In addition, the pain experienced is in the area of reproductive organs; therefore, it may not be surprising that such difficulties are common.

WOMEN'S OWN EXPERIENCES OF CARE FOR CHRONIC PELVIC PAIN

There is no doubt that chronic pelvic pain is associated with considerable ongoing distress. From a clinical perspective we need to understand the experiences of women with chronic pelvic pain and how services may be of best help to them. Understanding women's own perspectives are crucial in this process. Qualitative studies that have explored the woman's experience are rare but highly informative in this context. Savidge *et al.* have reported on a series of interviews with women with chronic pelvic pain who had a laparoscopy, where no abnormality was detected, between 12 and 18 months previously[18]. Almost all the women held specific beliefs about the causes of their pain, which often focused on the assumption of some physical damage from a reproductive event such as labor, miscarriage, termination or sterilization. A second category of explanation related the experience of life stressors, such as a bereavement or serious illness of a family member. These ideas were rarely explored by clinicians. The most valued aspects of the consultation with the GP centered around their listening, taking time to explain and showing concern and sympathy.

Following referral, women's expectations of the consultation with the gynecologist were typically high, focusing on gaining a solution to their pain. Only a quarter found these expectations realized and these women felt reassured by the information that there was nothing wrong. However, a majority of women were very dissatisfied about how information was relayed following the laparoscopy. Typically, they received information from a nurse or doctor, not previously met, some whilst still recovering from the anesthetic. There were obvious difficulties in processing information and having an opportunity to ask appropriate questions. Only a quarter received any medical follow-up. Explanations provided were either that there was no identifiable cause or that it might be a bowel problem. Whilst, as already stated, a quarter felt reassured, many expressed confusion/upset or anger and a feeling of not being taken seriously.

In terms of the ongoing impact, two-thirds were still experiencing pain 12–18 months later, and most reported an ongoing negative emotional impact together with adverse effects on several aspects of their lives including sexual activities, leisure and work. The summary of identified themes encapsulating their experience emphasized the need to ensure that others understood how much they hurt and did not dismiss their pain. The emotional impact was often intensified by a sense of not being believed and fueled by the sense of uncertainty generated by the lack of information. The final points concerned a sense of being helpless, isolated, coping alone and not knowing where to turn.

IMPLICATIONS FOR THE PROCESS OF CARE

In summary, women with chronic pelvic pain are likely to suffer considerable distress, not only in the experience of pain, but in terms of adverse effects on many aspects of their lives. It is crucial that in the initial discussions about the woman's pain, psychological and physical strands are considered together. This avoids the all too common scenario of a woman being referred to psychologists after multiple investigations have enhanced her belief in severity and pathology, leading to feelings of being 'fobbed-off' with distress unvalidated and disbelieved – this can be avoided by working closely with psychology in the initial stages of assessment, ideally within joint care clinics.

Recognizing the importance of the personal meanings of experienced symptoms and how these appraisals dramatically influence suffering and distress is crucial. Women also need explanations about how both physical and psychological mechanisms can interact in both the development and maintenance of pain, so that both sets of factors can be seen as relevant. There are obvious general implications relating to the process of care in the initial gynecological consultation in terms of the importance of professionals:

(1) Taking time to listen;

(2) Validating the experience of pain;

(3) Exploring and responding to women's own beliefs about causation;

(4) Providing educational materials indicating the fact that chronic pelvic pain is common and that clear explanations are sometimes unavailable;

(5) Being alert to the issues of sexual difficulties; and

(6) Being alert to the possibility of previous or current physical and/or sexual abuse.

After the operation there needs to be:

(1) Adequate time to recover from the anesthetic before being given feedback;

(2) A return appointment for clarification and questioning of explanations; and

(3) Where needed, a longer-term management plan.

Processes of care need to be organized to recognize the potential chronicity of the condition. It is important that the aim is management of difficulties, i.e. to reduce distress and increase quality of life rather than cure. Pain management programmes and mechanisms to reduce isolation and distress need to be developed to deal with the specific needs of chronic pelvic pain patients. These may incorporate cognitive behavioral strategies, which focus on the links between events, thoughts and feelings, and which may be particularly helpful in management. In addition, considering the role of fear of pain, hypervigilance and avoidance as factors in disability is also potentially valuable. Where previous sexual abuse appears to be a relevant factor in gynecological pain symptoms, an integrated psychological service would allow for appropriate care.

It is acknowledged that considering the possibility of sexual abuse within a gynecological consultation is not without its problems. Clinicians may feel inadequately skilled to deal with the sensitivity of the area and the possible information disclosed, and it may be difficult within the context of a busy clinic environment. Hence, there needs to be both adequate training and the facility to provide specialist follow-up care.

Working closely with psychology as an integrated part of the service for patients with chronic pelvic pain also allows for the training and support of staff around psychological aspects of care. It could also lead to simple screening processes for emotional distress relevant to presenting problems, as well as availability of brief integrated interventions as required.

The costs of inadequate attention to psychological factors are borne not only by the patient but by the clinic and its staff as well. For the service, this is likely to lead to the provision of repeated appointments, investigations and operations at very significant economic costs. Within the literature women have experienced up to 14 laparoscopies. For staff, work with this patient group may involve frequent experiences of frustration, helplessness and inadequacy, often mirroring the feelings of the women themselves.

To provide the most effective care, chronic pelvic pain needs to be considered within a clear integrated physical and psychological framework from the outset. Avoiding the trap identified by McGowan et al.[3], in which women become 'locked in a futile cycle of referral and investigation', is both clinically and economically desirable.

REFERENCES

1. Slade P, Anderton KJ, Faragher EB. Psychological aspects of gynaecological out-patients. J Psychosom Obstet Gynaecol 1988; 8: 77–94.

2. Slade P, Anderton KJ, Faragher EB. Psychological distress in gynaecological out-patients: cause or consequence. J Psychosom Obstet Gynaecol 1992; 13: 51–63.

3. McGowan L, Pitts M, Carter DC. Chronic pelvic pain: the general pactitioner's per-spective. Psychol Health Med 1999; 4: 303–17.

4. Slade P, Mathers N. 'An Unmet Need'. GP and Practice Nurse Perspectives on the Provision of Care for Psychological Issues related to Women's Reproductive Health. Report from the Institute of General Practice and Psychological Health, Sheffield, 2001.

5. Vlaeyen JWS, Linton SJ. Fear avoidance and its consequences in chronic muscu-loskeletal pain: a state of the art. Pain 2000; 85: 317–32.

6. Linton SJ, Buer N, Vlaeyen J, Hellsing AL. Are fear avoidance beliefs related to inception of an episode of back pain? A prospective study. Psychol Health 1999; 14: 1051–9.

7. Savidge C, Slade P. Psychological aspects of chronic pelvic pain. J Psychosom Res 1997; 42: 433–44.

8. Fry RPW, Beard RW, Crisp AH, McGuigan S. Sociopsychological factors in women with chronic pelvic pain with and without pelvic venous congestion. J Psychosom Res 1997; 42: 71–83.

9. Richter HE, Holley RL, Chandraiah S, Varner RE. Laparoscopic and psychologic evaluation of women with chronic pelvic pain. Int J Psychiatry Med 1998; 28: 243–53

10. Elcombe S, Gath D, Day A. The psychological effects of laparoscopy on women with chronic pelvic pain. Psychol Med 1999; 27: 1041–50.

11. Walker E, Katon W, Harrop-Griffiths J, et al. Relationship of chronic pelvic pain to psychiatric diagnoses and childhood sexual abuse. Am J Psychiatry 1988; 145: 75–80.

12. Reiter RC, Shakerin LR, Gambone DO, Milburn AK. Correlation between sexual abuse and somatization in women with somatic and non somatic chronic pelvic pain. Am J Obstet Gynecol 1991; 165: 104–9.

13. Rapkin AJ, Kames LD, Darke LL, et al. History of physical and sexual abuse in women with chronic pelvic pain. Obstet Gynecol 1990;76: 92–6.

14. Raphael KG, Widom CS, Lange G. Childhood victimization and pain in adulthood: a prospective investigation. Pain 2001; 92: 283–93.

15. Heim C, Ehlert U, Hanker JP, Hellhammer DH. Abuse-related posttraumatic stress disorder and alterations to the hypothalamic–pituitary–adrenal axis in women with chronic pelvic pain. Psychosom Med 1998; 60: 309–18.

16. Toomy TC, Hernandez JT, Gitterlman DF, Hulka JF. Relationship of sexual and physical abuse to pain and psychological assessment variables in chronic pelvic pain patients. Pain 1993; 53: 105–9.

17. Collett BJ, Cordle CJ, Stewart CR, Jagger C. A comparative study of women with chronic pelvic pain, chronic non-pelvic pain and no history of pain attending their GPs. Br J Obstet Gynaecol 1998; 105: 87–92.

18. Savidge C, Slade P, Stewart P, Li TC. Women's perspectives on their experiences of chronic pelvic pain and medical care. J Health Psychol 1998; 3: 103–16.

12

Unexplained pelvic pain

Hany Lashen

INTRODUCTION

Pelvic pain, defined as pain that originates or is felt in the pelvic or lower abdominal region, represents a challenge to clinicians across many disciplines. Gynecology, gastroenterology and urology are the disciplines in the forefront when dealing with pelvic pain. Psychiatrists and psychologists may also become involved at some point, since the complaint is often related to psychological and psychosomatic disorders. Acute pelvic pain is usually easier to deal with than chronic, non-specific pelvic pain.

In the absence of a defined pathological condition that can be objectively assessed, pelvic pain is often referred to as pelvic pain syndrome or unexplained pelvic pain (UPP). For the purpose of this article, UPP is the term that will be used as it is more informative and accurate since the condition does not have the requirements to qualify as a syndrome.

DEFINITION

As defined above, pelvic pain is any pain that is felt in or originates from the pelvis or lower abdomen. It can be acute as well as chronic. The chronicity of the condition increases the challenge faced by the clinician. Pelvic pain can also be cyclical in relation to or associated with a chronological event, such as menstruation (dysmenorrhea) or ovulation, or related to a physiological body function, such as intercourse (dyspareunia), micturition (dysuria) or defecation (dyschesia). Such association may offer a clue as to the origin of pain, which is often confused given the close proximity of the three main pelvic structures (rectum, bladder and reproductive organs). Other pelvic structures are often forgotten, such as the pelvic floor, the dysfunction of which can lead to chronic or even acute pelvic pain.

UPP can be defined as pain originating from or felt in the pelvis without an identifiable cause. Therefore, the diagnosis of UPP is only made by exclusion of all known causes.

CAUSES OF PELVIC PAIN

Having established that UPP can only be diagnosed by exclusion, knowledge of the various causes behind chronic pelvic pain is important. There are several ways to enumerate or classify the causes of pelvic pain. However, for the purpose of this chapter, the causes of pelvic pain will be considered under two main headings: gynecological and non-gynecological.

Gynecological causes of chronic pelvic pain

(1)   Primary dysmenorrhea;

(2)   Endometriosis;

(3)   Adenomyosis;

(4)   Pelvic inflammatory disease (PID);

(5)   Neoplasia, both benign and malignant;

(6)   Uterovaginal prolapse;

(7)   Less common causes:

    (a)   Residual ovary syndrome;

    (b)   Remnant ovary syndrome;

    (c)   Pelvic congestion syndrome;

    (d)   Postoperative adhesions.

Non-gynecological causes of chronic pelvic pain

These should include all urinary, intestinal and musculoskeletal causes.

Urinary causes

(1)   Urinary tract infection;

(2)   Urethral syndrome;

(3)   Urinary calculi;

(4)   Bladder cancer;

(5)   Detruser instability;

(6)   Voiding dysfunction;

(7)   Urinary retention.

Intestinal causes

(1)   Functional bowel disorders including irritable bowel syndrome (IBS). These conditions have been defined as chronic or recurrent symptoms for which there is no identifiable structural or biochemical cause, and include symptoms originating from the entire gastrointestinal tract[1]. IBS is the commonest of the functional bowel disorders as it affects 15–20% of the general population with more predilection toward women at a ratio of 2 : 1[2]. Prior to the introduction of specific diagnostic criteria, there was significant inconsistency in the reported figures of IBS epidemiology. A multinational working team decided on the diagnostic criteria, which they termed the Rome criteria[1]. These criteria were subsequently revised and called the Rome II criteria[1]. The Rome II criteria specify that the diagnosis of IBS can be made if, in the absence of structural or metabolic abnormalities for 12 weeks or more, in the past 12 months the patient complains of abdominal discomfort or pain that has two of the following features: relieved with defecation; onset associated with a change in frequency of stool; and onset associated with a change in form or appearance of stool. These were the essential criteria to make the diagnosis. However, there are other associated criteria that help strengthen the diagnosis[1]. Since the diagnosis of IBS requires the exclusion of an organic disease, the opinion of gastroenterologist colleagues is important if the condition is suspected. It is important, however, to remember that IBS can cause dyspareunia and that the symptoms can worsen during menses giving a false cyclical nature to the condition.

(2)   Proctalgia fugax – a benign, self-limiting pain experienced in the perineum. It is common, but most sufferers do not seek medical advice. The etiology is unclear, but a variation of IBS, pelvic floor myalgia and internal anal sphincter spasm have all been suggested. A careful history can elicit the characteristics, and simple reassurance is often all that is necessary. For persistent symptoms, therapies that induce internal anal sphincter relaxation are of value.

(3)   Diverticulitis. Diverticular disease is the commonest pathologic entity affecting the colon. It has been estimated to affect 35–50% of the population in the Western world. However, the incidence in patients younger than 40 years of age is approximately 5%.

(4)   Inflammatory bowel disease such as ulcerative colitis and Crohn's disease.

(5)   Malignancy.

Musculoskeletal causes

(1)   Lumbosacral displacement;

(2)   Osteoarthritis.

Psychological causes or elements

Women with chronic pelvic pain tend to have a relatively higher prevalence of depression and somatization. The incidence of childhood abuse and drug abuse is also high among such women. Other common symptoms found among women suffering from IBS, chronic pelvic pain and detrusor instability include anxiety and irritability. Many chronic conditions, especially if psychosomatic in nature, are made worse by stressful life events or the use of mind-altering drugs. It is essential, therefore, not to forget the impact the individual's psychology can have on the perception of disease and, unless such impact is palpable and easy to assess, efforts should be made to exclude somatic causes first. The issue of psychology will not be discussed further in this chapter; however, it should be mentioned that collaboration with psychiatric colleagues could prove tremendously helpful in assessing patients suffering from UPP.

DIAGNOSIS OF UNEXPLAINED PELVIC PAIN

To make this diagnosis all the aforementioned causes should be investigated and excluded. This requires a multidisciplinary team approach as well as robust diagnostic criteria. It may not always be easy to establish a multidisciplinary team in each hospital; therefore, reasonable links and communications should be established between gynecologists, urologists/urogynecologists and gastroenterologists/colorectal surgeons. I would even go so far as suggesting that failing to identify a reason for chronic pelvic pain warrants referral to a tertiary centre where the necessary expertise is available.

The key element in making the diagnosis, or at least for not missing a potentially treatable cause, is to adopt a systematic approach from the outset when dealing with patients presenting with pelvic pain. This will always start with careful history-taking by someone who is familiar with the potential causes of chronic pelvic pain and the diagnostic criteria for urological and gastroenterological as well as gynecological causes. Although at times the patient's history may be strongly suggestive of the cause, having preconceived ideas prior to starting the investigations can be detrimental to the clinician's effort in making the diagnosis and the doctor–patient relationship and rapport.

The commonest cause of UPP is a false-negative diagnosis. Therefore, and for practical reasons, the main emphasis in the remainder of this chapter will be on the potential pitfalls of diagnosis-making in patients presenting with chronic pelvic pain and addressing the treatment issue if the cause is not identifiable. To serve this purpose I would like to reclassify pelvic pain from a gynecologist's point of view into two main categories:

(1) Specific causes: these include endometriosis, PID and other neoplasia. If urogynecological causes are to be included under this section then all the urological causes should also be explored.

(2) Non-specific causes: these include pelvic congestion syndrome, residual ovary syndrome, remnant ovary syndrome, post-sterilization pelvic pain, and postoperative adhesions as a potential source of pelvic pain.

Furthermore, it is important at this point to mention that IBS and diverticular disease may co-exist with other gynecological conditions, which complicates the symptomatology and the patient's response to treatment. Therefore, these two conditions should be actively sought and excluded even in the presence of an obvious gynecological cause for the pain, especially in patients over 40 years of age.

Endometriosis

Endometriosis is discussed elsewhere in this book; however, a point of warning is that if endometriosis is suspected, a senior clinician's opinion should be considered in the absence of any obvious evidence of the condition on laparoscopy. The endometriotic lesions may present in different forms and shapes and other telltale signs may be all that are found on laparoscopy. Furthermore, adenomyosis cannot be diagnosed on laparoscopy and if the symptoms are strongly suggestive, magnetic resonance imaging (MRI) may prove useful and may save the patient an agonizing time undergoing other investigations. The severity of the condition as assessed visually does not correlate with the patient's symptomatology.

Pelvic congestion syndrome

Pelvic congestion syndrome is akin to varicocele in men. It is characterized by a dull aching pain due to reflux of blood in the dilated incompetent ovarian veins. This may lead to back pressure on the pampiniform plexus of veins in the broad ligament with obvious tortuous appearance at laparoscopy. The intensity of the pain is variable; however, the pain should persist for longer than 6 months in order to make the diagnosis. Sudden movements that lead to a sudden increase in abdominal pressure (e.g. bending or lifting heavy objects) exacerbate the pain. Usually the pain is unilateral and the condition is unique to multiparous women. Patients suffer from postcoital ache as well as dyspareunia. Other urinary complaints, perineal pain and dysmenorrhea have also been reported with this condition. Occasionally, vulval varicose veins may be visible. Ovarian point tenderness on abdominal examination has been suggested by Beard et al.[3] and Hobbs[4] as a characteristic clinical feature of the condition.

Diagnosis can be made by laparoscopy as well as imaging techniques, such as ultrasound and incremental and helical computed tomography scans. As the only reliable treatment in severe cases of this syndrome is total abdominal hysterectomy and bilateral salpingo-oophorectomy, the patient's favorable response to such a drastic option should be verified prior to embarking on surgery. Rendering the patient hypoestrogenemic using gonadotropin-releasing hormone (GnRH) analogs or long-term progestogen therapy would be advisable. Improvement in the patient's symptoms is a reasonable indication that she should benefit from the operation. In milder cases, the use of progestogens alone may prove useful. However, there are specific causes of pelvic congestion syndrome that should be investigated, such as the nutcracker syndrome[5]; this could be treated without having to resort to total abdominal hysterectomy and bilateral salpingo-oophorectomy.

Residual ovary syndrome

Occasionally, women who have undergone total abdominal hysterectomy for menstrual flow problems may return with pelvic pain that some assign to the ovaries that were left behind. This is known as residual ovary syndrome. In many cases, the pain is physiological due to ovulation and follicle development in an anchored ovary. Occasionally, the ovary will become entrapped in adhesions, particularly in the vaginal vault, and be the source of pain, which is usually cyclical, but it may also cause dyspareunia. Although this condition is relatively rare, oophorectomy is often required to bring relief to the patient from her symptoms.

Ovarian remnant syndrome

Ovarian remnant syndrome usually arises in endometriosis patients who continue to suffer from cyclical pelvic pain after removal of both ovaries. Ovarian tissue that is left behind during a difficult surgery autografts itself to other tissues, especially the bowels or mesentery, and continues to produce estrogen in a cyclical fashion. If that tissue contained residual endometriosis, it can potentially lead to the development of an endometriotic cyst, which is less responsive to GnRH agonist treatment. This condition is very rare, and I personally have come across only two cases in my professional career. A lack of or mild menopausal symptoms despite not taking hormone replacement therapy may be a clue to the presence of ovarian remnants. The persistence of premenstrual syndrome symptoms may also be another clue. The development of *de novo* cyclical bowel symptoms may be due to implantation of the ovarian endometriotic tissue in the bowel. An MRI scan may be useful in alerting the clinician to the diagnosis; however, in most cases, a laparotomy and careful systematic inspection of the abdomen may be necessary. Removal of the ovarian remnants is expected to lead to a dramatic improvement in most patients.

Post-sterilization pelvic pain and postoperative pelvic adhesions

Tubal sterilization is the commonest procedure worldwide. Despite the overall satisfaction and low side-effects, some patients report abdominal pain and menstrual problems that follow the procedure. This has led to the emergence of the term 'post-tubal sterilization syndrome'. This syndrome includes pain and irregular bleeding as well as psychosexual symptoms and an increase in the frequency of premenstrual symptoms. It is not known whether such a syndrome really exists, as it affects only a small number of women and there is no evidence about the influence of other confounding variables. If it does exist it affects a minority of women; however, given the wide scale of tubal sterilization the number can soon become significant enough for the average gynecologist to come across some cases. There are several reports of abdominal and pelvic pain due to detachment of the Filshie clip and its implantation somewhere else in the abdomen and pelvis.

Postoperative adhesions, defined as fibrous connections that may contain vascular channels which join tissue surfaces in abnormal locations[6] have received increasing attention owing to potential complications. Adhesions are known to cause small bowel obstruction and infertility. However, chronic pain and organ dysfunction including the bowel and other pelvic organs do not receive wide support. Despite the controversy over whether adhesions cause pain, Duffy and diZerega[7] reported 60–90% improvement in symptoms after adhesiolysis. Discussing pelvic adhesion in detail is beyond the remit of this chapter; however, the author believes that dense adhesions that restrict an organ's mobility may lead to pain. Adhesiolysis can relieve the symptoms in many cases, but, given the adhesions' tremendous propensity to reform, the pain relief may be short lived and the clinician should endeavor in these cases to use adhesion prevention barriers.

In conclusion, the accuracy and frequency of diagnosing UPP depends on the clinician's experience as well as his/her knowledge of the different causes of pelvic pain and the availability of a multidisciplinary team to consult with prior to excluding all known causes of chronic pelvic pain. UPP is not an easy diagnosis for the patients to accept for reasons that are discussed below. Therefore, every effort should be made to exclude all potential known causes and to have a plan of management in cases of UPP. Establishing a rapport with the patient from the outset can be very valuable in dealing with the patient, having offered her no specific diagnosis.

PROBLEMS ASSOCIATED WITH UNEXPLAINED PELVIC PAIN

Chronic pelvic pain is generally a protracted condition that has a psychological impact on the patient and her family, work and social life. Furthermore, patients' expectations are very high, and with sufficient knowledge available on the Internet the clinician should be extremely up-to-date when dealing with these patients. Such expectations no doubt put pressure on health workers dealing with patients presenting with chronic pelvic pain. The situation is usually better for the patient and easier to accept if a specific diagnosis is made, otherwise under the psychological pressure the patient will tend to doubt herself, which may lead to more psychological morbidity.

MANAGEMENT OF UNEXPLAINED PELVIC PAIN

Non-specific conditions require non-specific treatments that are usually empirical with one main objective – to improve the quality of life for the patient. Most of the available treatment modalities have not been the subject of randomized controlled trials, which limits the strength of the supporting evidence. Furthermore, carrying out of such trials may prove impossible due to diagnostic difficulties and potential variation in the underlying pathology, if any, in patients with UPP. In addition, the number of patients seen with this condition is relatively small, so not all gynecologists can develop the skills and necessary expertise to deal with these patients, not to mention establish a multidisciplinary team. The available treatment modalities and some advice on the management of UPP are the subjects of this section.

Before discussing treatments I would like to reiterate the importance of two points with regard to diagnosis:

(1)   It should be endeavoured to make a diagnosis or at least not to miss a diagnosis and remembered that an identifiable cause is easier for the clinician to treat and for the patient to accept. Missing an identifiable cause may have serious medicolegal consequences, as well as resulting in disappointment for the patient.

(2)   Multidisciplinary team approach: once the specific and non-specific gynecological reasons have been excluded, the clinician will be left with different possibilities including the patient's psyche. Inviting the relevant expertise

may lead to identification of a previously unrecognized etiology or patholo-gy, or at least exclude it from the equation. Despite a lack of evidence, I believe that a team approach is easier and friendlier for the patient com-pared with a series of referrals from one specialist to another. A team approach will reduce the patient's anxiety and confusion, which can result from hearing different explanations, and is unlikely to affect the continuity of care.

As mentioned above, 'non-specific' is the key word here and some treatment modalities may help establish the cause. The modalities of treatment that can be offered fall into the following categories.

Medical management

Suppression of gonadal function using gonadotropin-releasing hormone agonists or progestogens

This will help the clinician to evaluate the impact of sex steroids and the changes around the menstrual cycle, both physiological and psychological, in terms of the intensity and perception of pain. A significant improvement would indicate that gonadal suppression should be part of the treatment strategy. Nonetheless, con-tinuing this treatment for at least a year prior to contemplating offering the patient a permanent solution, such as a hysterectomy, is advisable; this is to allow for adjustment on behalf of the patient and for proper evaluation of the response. To avoid the unwanted effects of GnRH agonists on the bones and back, hormone replacement therapy should be offered.

General advice on the management of constipation and other non-specific bowel dysfunction, or even empirical treatment for IBS, may prove useful. Two randomized controlled trials[8] have explored the value of a progestogen (medroxy-progesterone acetate) in the treatment of unexplained chronic pelvic pain. The evidence indicates that while on treatment chronic pelvic pain sufferers show improvement in their symptoms, which recur upon discontinuation of the medications.

Analgesics

Analgesics are an easy approach to take in order to improve the patient's quality of life. However, such treatment should be part of a strategy that includes ade-quate psychological support via counseling or cognitive therapy. Advice from the pain clinic on the control and strategy of analgesic therapy in patients with UPP ought to be sought.

Antidepressants

The use of antidepressants in the management of a variety of conditions associated with chronic pain has demonstrated some benefit. This may be due to the complex nature of the individual's perception of pain or to the higher prevalence of psychological disorders among chronic pain sufferers. In a prospective, double-blind, placebo-controlled crossover study, Engel et al. reported the lack of a significant improvement in pain or functional disability on sertraline, compared with placebo[9]. However, the study included a small number of patients and the main outcome measure was intensity of pain after 6 weeks of sertraline therapy. These two points limit the value of the study and restrict its conclusion on the efficacy of antidepressants. However, this remains the only prospective randomized trial available addressing this issue.

Psychological assessment and counseling

Again, this is a non-specific treatment or support offered to all patients with chronic conditions that affect their quality of life. Psychosexual counseling may prove beneficial in some cases where dyspareunia is the primary complaint. As numerous studies[10] have reported a higher rate of childhood and adult abuse among chronic pelvic pain sufferers, both physical and sexual, the need for psychological counseling and assessment is paramount. Most clinicians will not be trained or qualified to investigate or unravel such a possibility and enlisting the help of psychologists and psychiatrists may prove priceless.

Surgical management

Common sense and traditional good medical teachings alert us to the value of not embarking on surgical treatment for unknown conditions. Furthermore, a significant part of patients' counseling on the value of any treatment should also include the implications, as well as complications, that may arise from the suggested treatment. Strictly speaking, this cannot be said about surgery for UPP. Offering a hysterectomy for UPP is a gamble that may prove more devastating for the patient, particularly psychologically.

Role of the pain clinic

The pain clinic has a lot to offer not only with regard to treatment but also in investigating the cause.

Complementary and alternative medicine

The evidence for such treatment is certainly not forthcoming or even available. Alternative medicine is not subject to the same rigorous measurements applied to medical treatments. However, some evidence is emerging on the value of acupuncture in medicine, which is encouraging. Selecting the route of alternative medicine is the patient's choice and medics are unable to offer negative or positive advice due to lack of evidence.

REFERENCES

1. Thompson WG, Creed F, Drossman DA, et al. Functional bowel disorders and chronic functional abdominal pain. Gastroenterol Int 1992; 5: 75–91.

2. Talley NJ, Zinmeister AR, Van Dyke C, Melton LJ 3rd. Epidemiology of colonic symptoms and the irritable bowel syndrome. Gastroenterology 1991; 101: 927–34.

3. Beard RW, Reginald PW, Wadsworth J. Clinical features of women with chronic lower abdominal pain and pelvic congestion. Br J Obstet Gynaecol 1988; 5: 153–61.

4. Hobbs JT. The pelvic congestion syndrome. Br J Hosp Med 1990; 43: 199–206.

5. Scultetus AH, Villavicencio JL, Gillespie DL. The nutcracker syndrome: its role in the pelvic venous disorders. J Vasc Surg 2001; 34: 812–19.

6. Diamond MP. Incidence of postsurgical adhesions. In diZerega G, ed. Peritoneal Surgery. New York: Springer-Verlag, 2000: 217–20.

7. Duffy DM, diZerega GS. Adhesions controversies: pelvic pain as a cause of adhesions, crystalloids in preventing them. J Reprod Med 1996; 41: 19–26.

8. Farquhar CM, Rogers V, Franks S, et al. A randomised controlled trial of medroxyprogesterone acetate and psychotherapy for the treatment of pelvic congestion. Br J Obstet Gynaecol 1989; 96: 1153–62.

9.   Engel C, Walker EA, Engel AL, Armstrong A. A randomised, double blind crossover trial of sertraline in women with chronic pelvic pain. J Psychsom Res 1998; 44: 203–7.

10. Soysal ME, Soysal S, Vicdan K, Ozer S. A randomised controlled trial of goserlin and medroxyprogesterone acetate in the treatment of pelvic congestion. Hum Reprod 2001; 16: 931–9.

13

Pelvic pain clinic: a multidisciplinary approach

Cornelia CT Wiesender

INTRODUCTION

Chronic pelvic pain is a difficult problem. It is not a disease but a complex syndrome, which is often frustrating for the patient and clinician. With a prevalence similar to asthma and back pain it is highly significant; 10% of gynecological outpatient consultations are for pelvic pain[1], yet these only represent a highly selected subgroup. A large number of women with chronic pelvic pain (60%) are not referred or given a diagnosis by their general practitioner[2].

Most patients go through a lengthy and depressing journey from specialist to specialist in search for a cause and cure, and many have undergone multiple operations without long-term benefit. The traditional medical approach has not proven to be successful in patients with chronic pelvic pain. The pelvic pain clinic is based on the concept of a multidisciplinary approach, which acknowledges the multifactorial nature of the problem and aims to help the patient understand and manage her symptoms better.

WHAT IS A MULTIDISCIPLINARY APPROACH?

The multidisciplinary approach incorporates several healthcare professionals from different specialities. They work together in a team. This is in contrast to one practitioner referring to other specialists as and when needed. The group assesses, evaluates and decides on the management of the patient together. The great advantage of such an approach is that it emphasizes to the patient and family the multifactorial nature of the pain and the importance of all aspects of it. This approach makes it very clear for the patient that all members of the team are equally important.

REASONS FOR A MULTIDISCIPLINARY APPROACH

The management of chronic pelvic pain remains a difficult problem in terms of both its diagnosis and treatment. The pathophysiology of chronic pelvic pain is poorly understood. Two neurophysiological mechanisms are implicated: nociceptive pain, which is somatic or visceral in origin, or non-nociceptive pain, which is neuropathic or psychogenic[3]. It is also important to consider the interactions that occur between the reproductive organs and urinary and gastrointestinal tracts[5]. To complicate matters further, inflammation or congestion of the reproductive organs can be physiological from ovulation or menstruation. This explains menstrual exacerbation of chronic pelvic pain. However, in many women with chronic pelvic pain no pathology has been found. Approximately 40% of laparoscopies performed for pelvic pain are negative[4]. In these cases the cause of pain is often thought to be psychogenic. The assumption that pain has to be linked with some form of pathology is not helpful. Unfortunately the dichotomy inherent in the Cartesian theory of pain – either organic or psychological – is widely accepted. The problem, however, is more complex and it is more likely that a number of factors are causing and contributing to the pain. The biopsychosocial model takes this into account and allows a broader approach. Reiter[5] claims that chronic pelvic pain is best understood as resulting from a complex interrelationship between sensory stimulation (neurologic, musculoskeletal, endocrine), psychological factors and socioenvironmental factors, whereby each of these components is capable of influencing the others.

The traditional approach to this disorder has been surgical: 30–40% of laparoscopies and 10–12% of hysterectomies are performed for chronic pelvic pain, although the long-term outcome has been disappointing[6–8]. This is perhaps not surprising as it is also well known that where pathology such as endometriosis, adhesions or pelvic inflammatory disease is present, the severity often poorly correlates with the extent of the pain[9].

A multidisciplinary treatment approach has been shown to be more effective than unimodal treatment for chronic pain conditions.[10] The International Association for the Study of Pain provides scientific evidence that chronic pain is a biopsychosocial event and that its diagnosis and treatment should be considered in a multidisciplinary frame[11]. In such a team a complete, simultaneous assessment can be made where each component is mapped and a holistic diagnosis is reached.

Guzman *et al.* performed a review of the Cochrane Database (2002) on the treatment of chronic low back pain. This has revealed strong evidence that multidisciplinary biopsychosocial rehabilitation with a functional restoration approach improves function and pain when compared with non-multidisciplinary treatments. The evidence for vocational outcomes (return to work and sickness leave) was contradictory between the trials[12]. This approach has been adapted for chronic pelvic pain and the major evidence to support a multidisciplinary approach comes from a randomized trial by Peters *et al.*[13]. This paper showed an advantage of the multidisciplinary approach vs. conventional management in quality-of-life outcomes, but not the McGill pain score. Gambone and Reiter showed that the introduction of a multidisciplinary approach not only led to symptomatic improvement but also to a reduction in the hysterectomy rate from approximately 15–20% to 6%[14]. Stones and Price concluded from a review of chronic pelvic pain referrals to pain clinics that women with chronic pelvic pain seemed to be referred considerably less than those with chronic musculoskeletal pain[15]. They assumed that the reasons for this were that some women were still searching for a cure and that participation in group activities can be difficult because of the intimate nature of the problem.

THE PELVIC PAIN CLINIC

The pelvic pain clinic was established by three different specialists with a particular interest in pelvic pain: a gynecologist, an anesthetist specializing in pain management and a clinical psychologist.

This team conducts the consultation and initial assessment of the patient. Although a physiotherapist and a clinical nurse specialist should ideally be present, many patients would find a large number of healthcare specialists threatening. Close liaison with a gastroenterologist, a urologist, an orthopedic surgeon and a psychiatrist with an interest in pain problems is important. Sometimes patients may need to be referred for another specialist's opinion.

Patients are referred to the pelvic pain clinic for secondary and tertiary care. Nevertheless most referrals from primary care have been seen by at least one specialist previously. At present, resources allow us to run this clinic only once a month and overall access to multidisciplinary pain clinics in the UK is limited, which means primary referrals can only rarely be seen and some form of selection has to take place. This selection is usually based on the severity of the pain and an unsatisfactory response to conventional gynecological treatment. The aims of the clinic are clearly established: they are to assess all aspects of the patient's symptoms and their impact on the patient's life carefully and, from there, to relieve the pain but most importantly reduce the physical and emotional dysfunction, help the patient to develop coping strategies and so improve quality of life.

An information booklet about the clinic is sent to the patient prior to the appointment. This booklet gives some information on chronic pelvic pain and describes the nature of the clinic, the procedure, the personnel involved and its goals. Together with the booklet the patient receives a questionnaire and a pain diary, which she is asked to complete ideally over at least a 2-month period prior to the clinic appointment. This is useful for data collection and auditing, but may also help with history-taking.

Because of the nature of the clinic about 45–60 minutes' consultation time is needed for each patient. It is important that the patient is informed about this well in advance in order to make the appropriate arrangements, otherwise a rushed consultation may be unsatisfactory. As such a clinic set-up, with multiple clinicians, can be intimidating, the patient is encouraged to be accompanied by their partner, a close relative or friend. It is essential that she sees the positive aspects of such a set-up and feels at ease.

The advantage of such a clinic is that the patient has to tell her story only once and it can be heard by all members of the team. Most patients have a long string of consultations and multiple story-telling can be frustrating. The patient is assessed holistically, taking a full medical, social, psychological and sexual history. All members of the team are equally contributing to this assessment. It is crucially important, however, that the patient does not feel threatened or 'on trial'. Instead she should feel that this is an opportunity to voice all her feelings and concerns.

As part of the initial assessment it is important to establish the patient's goals and expectations. Some patients simply want an explanation for the cause of the pain, whereas others wish for symptom control or hope for cure. Sometimes patients feel this is an opportunity to receive clarification about diagnoses, investigations and treatments received in the past. The patient's satisfaction of the consultation depends very much on these initial expectations. A good initial consultation has been shown to have a favorable outcome especially in those patients without exercise impairment[15].

A full examination is necessary. This includes abdominal, and sometimes neurological examinations and assessment of posture/back. Although most patients have seen a gynecologist before, a gynecological examination is almost always necessary, not so much to identify pathology but to locate tender areas and assess for muscle spasm and vaginismus.

After this initial assessment, the team will make an evaluation and decide on the treatment while the patient is asked to wait outside the consultation room. A full explanation of the impression and proposed treatment needs to be given to the patient and accompanying person.

Part of the treatment may be referral to a woman's health physiotherapist or further assessment/management by one or more members of the team. Some patients will be enrolled in a multidisciplinary pain management programme. Follow-up in the multidisciplinary clinic is rarely needed and should be discussed carefully as repeated follow-up may lead to increased patient expectations and to a medicalization of symptoms. Instead a pelvic pain support group can be helpful for a number of patients. In such a group the ongoing needs that go beyond the scope of routine hospital and clinic appointments may be met. Not all find it easy to talk about intimate problems in a group but a lot of patients feel very alone and alienated with their symptoms, in which case a support group can be useful. We have initiated such a group recently following experience from the pelvic pain clinic. A clinical psychologist provides input into this support group and acts as a link. The objectives of the support group are to help patients develop a positive and proactive approach to managing their pain, to gain support and understanding from others in a similar situation and to help reduce the impact of pain on their daily life.

The patient's general practitioner (GP) will be informed about the consultation, and the patient will receive a copy of this letter. Any sensitive issues the patient does not wish to be disclosed to the GP will remain confidential. As some patients who attend the pelvic pain clinic have been referred from a different health authority, treatment recommendations have to be made clearly within this letter and referral, for example to a psychologist or women's health physiotherapist, will have to be arranged by the initial referrer.

We do not include a nurse specialist in our team because of the team size, as mentioned before. Perhaps this will change in the future depending on further research but clearly any changes in the team need to be considered very carefully. A nurse specialist could provide valuable input into the team by acting as a point of contact for the patient and for this purpose operate a helpline. Any questions arising after the consultation could be discussed with the nurse in a non-threatening environment. Some patients feel more comfortable discussing certain topics with a nurse rather than a doctor. Chronic pelvic pain patients often have repeated acute hospital admissions. In such cases the nurse specialist could liaise between the ward staff and the multidisciplinary team. The nurse can also provide education for the ward staff on the complexity of chronic pelvic pain.

THE ROLES OF THE INDIVIDUAL TEAM MEMBERS

The gynecologist

The role of the gynecologist is multifactorial. In some patients treatable disease may not have been diagnosed yet. However, the majority of patients who are referred to the pelvic pain clinic have had their symptoms for many months or years and have been seen by a number of gynecologists and/or other specialists. They have had various investigations and most patients have undergone a number of unsuccessful medical and surgical interventions. They would have received one or more diagnoses. Not only has the pain not been cured but often they are now also experiencing post-surgical neuropathic pain. This unsatisfactory process has often increased the patient's anxiety and worries which, in turn, can exacerbate the symptoms. It is well recognized that pain perception is modulated by fear, depression and anxiety[16]. Despite (or because of) many patients having this long trail of specialists, diagnosis and treatment, they have a confused picture about what is wrong with them or what has happened to them and are desperate for clarification.

The conventional medical approach is to investigate the symptoms, make a diagnosis and institute treatment, which hopefully leads to cure. This approach has not been helpful with chronic pelvic pain probably because of the more complex nature of the problem. Laparoscopy is claimed to be the gold standard in gynecolocial investigations for pelvic pain but it is important to remember that many disorders contribute to chronic pelvic pain that cannot be diagnosed by the laparoscope[5,13]. The prevalence and type of pathology found at laparoscopy tends to vary between studies and is significantly higher in the surgical research groups, compared with the psychologically oriented groups[17]. It is not clear whether pathological findings such as endometriosis, pelvic inflammatory disease or adhesions are the cause of the patient's symptoms, and yet this is often conveyed to the patient with undoubtable certainty. In particular, endometriosis is well recognized as having a paradoxical appearance. It is detected in 44–49% of asymptomatic women. About 50% of women with documented disease do not complain of pain[17,18], whereas others with minimal findings are given an irrefutable diagnosis for the cause of their symptoms. Equally, those with the same symptoms but a negative laparoscopy are dismissed.

Once a diagnosis is made, the patient and doctor get trapped in the expectation of cure. Therefore, making a diagnosis is not always helpful. The role of the gynecologist within the pelvic pain clinic is to break this cycle and fixation on diagnosis and cure. The patient may have to accept that cure is not always possible and that her goals should shift towards symptom relief and pain management. Also, there is usually more than one factor responsible for the woman's symptoms and surgical approaches have been overemphasized. As Peters *et al.* put it: 'The tendency among gynecologists to select a surgical approach to the problem appears to be related to the values and specific functions that are attributed to the organs that can be removed. There is a tendency to limit the importance of internal genital organs to their reproductive function and thus to consider them largely superfluous after that function has been fulfilled'[13].

In the multidisciplinary clinic, the gynecologist is trying to find an explanation and point out to the patient the multifactorial cause for her symptoms. It is important to provide an explanation for the symptoms, interventions and diagnoses made so far. This can ease the patient's reorientation from a search for cure towards pain management. Patients who still believe there is a cure lack the high motivation required for strategies such as cognitive behavioral therapy.

Apart from taking a normal history, it is important to identify events that coincided with the first occurrence of the pain and events that lead to an exacerbation or improvement. The relationship of symptoms to the menstrual cycle can be important because functional events can exacerbate pain. These can often be improved with hormonal manipulation. A decision has to be made whether more investigations are required although this is rarely necessary. Some symptoms are related to the loss or fear of fertility. This can be clarified within the team and the benefit of appropriate investigations or surgery evaluated.

The psychologist

The International Association for the Study of Pain recommends that a clinical psychologist should be included in a chronic pelvic pain team and the significance of this is well documented in the literature[19]. The importance of psychological variables and how they can affect the reaction to pain was first formulated by Melzack in 1965 in his 'gate control theory of pain'[20]. With chronic pain in particular, successful pain control often involves changing the cognitive–motivational components while the sensory component remains intact.

The advantage of the psychologist being present at the first assessment is that he/she can be introduced as an equal member of the team and as someone who can help with his/her special expertise. Pain patients are typically suspicious of a psychologist as they perceive their problem as physical and may be worried that doctors believe 'it is all in their head'. The false duality between physical and psychological is well established among lay people and health professionals, although there is much evidence that both are closely interrelated in all aspects of pain detection, transmission and perception. It is therefore essential to avoid any discussion about physical or mental, but instead stress their close relationship and that the psychologist has special training to help the patient coping with the effects the pain has on her life.

It is important to be aware of any past psychiatric history. Many studies have shown that women with chronic pelvic pain have high levels of anxiety, depression/low mood and anger[21]. Mood disorders can affect pain intensity and prevent motivation for a self-management approach. It does not matter whether the patient has been found to have a pathology, e.g. endometriosis, or not; the likelihood of a mood disorder is the same[15]. Also, these patients often feel a loss of control, which can exacerbate their pain.

Various studies have shown that women with chronic pelvic pain have a higher lifetime prevalence of sexual abuse[22]. This association does not imply causality but an awareness of the association is important. The psychologist needs to make a thorough psychosocial and behavioral assessment, although some topics may provoke extreme distress and therefore deeper questioning may have to be deferred for a separate session.

Grace argues that the psychogenic effect as a cause of pain is underrated[23]. However, these notions about 'organic' vs. 'psychological' pain are counterproductive and a step forward would be to accept the limitations in current knowledge about the etiology of chronic pelvic pain. It is essential for the pelvic pain patient that she does not feel that doctors believe there is nothing wrong with her.

Furthermore, psychological stress often manifests itself as somatic symptoms and it is well known that chronic pelvic pain patients have more somatic symptoms than patients without pain[22]. Kamm uses the biopsychosocial model and asserts that 'specific physiological mechanisms must link psychological events with altered somatic function such as altered bowel function, pelvic venous dilatation or increased visceral sensitivity'[23].

The role of the psychologist is to identify any 'stressors' and factors contributing to or exacerbating the pain. He/she should explore the patient's feelings, expectations and worries about the pain and what impact it has on her life and sexual relationship. The prevalence of sexual problems is much higher in this group[22]. A psychosexual assessment is therefore very important. The woman's needs and her coping mechanisms are explored. From there a special pain management programme can be developed, which may include stress management (relaxation techniques, self-hypnosis), assertiveness and communication skills training, pacing and activity scheduling, cognitive behavioral therapy techniques and psychosexual therapy. The primary aim of the latter is to break the pain–dysfunction–pain cycle. Cognitive strategies attempt to change the way patients think about pain and to increase the patient's feeling of control over all aspects of the problem.

The anesthetist

Most of the doctors involved in providing pain management services are anesthetists who have undergone specialist training in this field. They are familiar with the biopsychosocial model of pain and accustomed to working within a multidisciplinary team. Chronic pelvic pain is similar to many other chronic pain conditions and therefore an anesthetist who is familiar with the concept of symptom management is a valuable member of the team. He/she can be very helpful in the initial assessment of the patient and evaluation of the type of pain, which can be chronic somatic, visceral or neuropathic.

The anesthetist's expertise in the prescription of analgesic drugs can be of great value as many patients are using or have tried a number of analgesics. Certain chronic pains, especially neuropathic pain, respond well to drugs that are not typical analgesics, such as tricyclic antidepressants (e.g. amitriptyline, imipramine), anti-convulsants (e.g. carbamazepine, gabapentin) and membrane-stabilizing drugs (e.g. mexiletine). These drugs, if used for pain management, often require specific dosages and the anesthetist will be familiar with these.

Anesthetists have the ability to perform diagnostic, prognostic and therapeutic nerve blockades and are accustomed to alternative treatments such as acupuncture or transcutaneous electrical nerve stimulation.

A careful examination of the patient may reveal skeletal structures of the spine or pelvis such as facet joints or the sacroiliac joint producing referred pain, which is perceived as visceral pain. In such cases therapeutic facet joint injections with a long-acting steroid may be considered.

Pain evokes muscle tension, which in return exacerbates the pain[16]. The role of musculoskeletal dysfunction as a cause of chronic pelvic pain is well documented[21]. There may be direct trauma, such as accidents, childbirth or surgery, but more commonly musculoskeletal problems are a result of chronic strain associated with poor posture and poor physical fitness. Pain from musculoskeletal structures of the back and pelvis can mimic pain of gynecological or urological origin and vary in intensity throughout the menstrual cycle due to hormonal changes, which can compound diagnostic confusion[24]. The anesthetist with a special interest in pain management is well trained to identify these problems and referral to a physiotherapist can be initiated.

Trigger points may be identified. These are small hypersensitive regions within the muscle or fascia. On compression they can give rise to referred pain. Trigger points may be in the abdominal wall, vaginal vault or pelvic floor musculature. They can be injected with a long-acting local anesthetic; alternatively, treatment with physiotherapy has been shown to be helpful.

The physiotherapist has an important role in the management of chronic pelvic pain, although we feel that he/she need not be present at the initial consultation. As mentioned before, too large a number of health professionals could be intimidating for the patient. A close relationship with a women's health physiotherapist is very important.

AUDIT/OUTCOME MEASURES

To assess the value of such a clinic and justify the implications on resources, it is important to audit/monitor the outcome. The outcome measures need to be clearly related to the aims of the clinic. Pain intensity can be analyzed by using a numerical or visual analog self-rating scale. There are more objective ways of assessing the patient's progress, for example use of medication or alternative treatments, number of hospital admissions, number of GP visits or consultation with further specialists. It is an important aim of the multidisciplinary clinic to reduce the use of healthcare services.

How the patient is coping with her symptoms is an important outcome measure and can be analyzed with a numerical scale.

Quality-of-life improvement can be assessed with specific measures such as social and sexual function using a standardized questionnaire. Another outcome measure could be return to work. However, this is hard to apply in this group as many women may have chosen not to work in the first place. To make improvements it is necessary to evaluate the patient's satisfaction with the clinic visit and identify aspects she liked or disliked.

All the patients seen in the pelvic pain clinic receive a questionnaire after 6 months and 1 year. This includes most of the outcome measures mentioned above. It is difficult, however, to analyze these data as we see a very heterogeneous group in our clinic, and patients who receive treatment within the health authority may have different outcomes than those referred from other health authorities where close liaison with team members and other healthcare professionals involved in the woman's care is not easily possible.

RESEARCH AND EDUCATION

There are only a few multidisciplinary clinics for chronic pelvic pain and more research is required to assess this approach and how it should develop. Research is also needed to clarify which elements are important in the patient's experience and which health professionals should be included in the multidisciplinary team.

It is uncertain whether such a clinic should function as a tertiary referral setting or whether a totally different approach should be adopted, whereby patients are referred after the first recurrence of the pain, before they have undergone the cycle of multiple investigations and failed treatments. Future studies may show that it would be better if the woman could be seen in a multidisciplinary pelvic pain clinic early on to prevent progression into the chronic pain state. Peters *et al.* have already shown in a study from 1991 that better outcome was achieved if there was equal attention both to organic and other causative factors from the beginning of therapy than with a standard approach[13].

The pelvic pain clinic is a valuable teaching opportunity for students and all professionals involved in the care of women. However, increasing the number of professionals in the clinic is not helpful for making the patient feel at ease. This could be helped by the use of video screening with the patient's permission.

As chronic pelvic pain is a common and often frustrating problem, it should be given more attention in the undergraduate curriculum. Consulting styles that address the patient's needs for explanation rather than pursuit of a pathological diagnosis, and communication skills required to convey diagnostic uncertainty or negative findings without undermining the patient's confidence, need to be part of medical education[25].

CONCLUSIONS

Chronic pelvic pain is a complex condition that has frustrated many clinicians and patients. The conventional unimodal approach fixed on diagnosis–treatment–cure has not proved to be successful. Because of the multifactorial nature of the problem, a multidisciplinary approach which is used in the pelvic pain clinic appears to be more effective. The patient can be assessed and treated using the biopsychosocial concept, which sees the patient in a holistic way. However, there is still potential for development and an increased understanding is required as to which health professionals should be included in the team. Further research is needed to elicit the important elements of the clinic to achieve the best outcome for the patient.

REFERENCES

1. Reiter RC. A profile of women with chronic pelvic pain. Clin Obstet Gynecol 1990; 33: 130–6.

2. Zondervan KT, Yudkin PL, Vessey MP, et al. The prevalence of chronic pelvic pain in women in the United Kingdom: a systematic review. Br J Obstet Gynaecol 1998; 105: 93-9.

3. Gunter J. Chronic pelvic pain: an integrated approach to diagnosis and treatment. Obstet Gynecol Surv 2003; 58: 615–23.

4. Moore J, Kennedy S. Causes of chronic pelvic pain. Bailliere's Best Pract Res Clin Obstet Gynaecol 2000; 14: 389–402.

5. Reiter RC. Evidence-based management of chronic pelvic pain. Clin Obstet Gynecol 1998; 41: 422–35.

6.   Howard FM. The role of laparoscopy in chronic pelvic pain: promise and pitfalls. Obstet Gynecol Surv 1993; 48: 357–87.

7.   Dicker RC, Greenspan JR, Straus LT, et al. Complications of abdominal and vaginal hysterectomy among women of reproductive age in the United States. Am J Obstet Gynecol 1992; 144: 841–8.

8.   Lee NC, Dicker RC, Rubin GL, et al. Confirmation of the preoperative diagnosis for hysterectomy. Am J Obstet Gynecol 1984; 150: 283–7.

9.   Rapkin AJ. Adhesions and pelvic pain: a retrospective study. Obstet Gynecol 1986; 68: 13–15.

10.   Flor H, Fydrich T, Turk DC. Efficacy of multidisciplinary pain treatment centers: a meta-analysis review. Pain 1992; 49: 221–30.

11.   Poppe C, Devulder J, Mariman A, Mortier E. Chronic pain therapy: an evolution from solo-interventions to a holistic interdisciplinary patient approach. Acta Clin Belg 2003; 58: 92–7.

12.   Guzman J, Esmail R, Karjalainen K, et al. Multidisciplinary bio-psycho-social rehabilitation for chronic low back pain. Evid Base Nurs 2002; 5: 116.

13.   Peters AAW, Dorst E, Jellis B, et al. A randomized clinical trial to compare two different approaches in women with chronic pelvic pain. Obstet Gynecol 1991; 77: 740–4.

14.   Gambone JC, Reiter RC. Nonsurgical management of chronic pelvic pain: a multidisciplinary approach. Clin Obstet Gynecol 1990; 33: 205–11.

15.   Stones RW, Price C. Health services for women with chronic pelvic pain. J R Soc Med 2002; 95: 531–5.

16.   Newton-John T. The psychology of pain. In MacLean AB, Stones RW, Thornton S, eds. Pain in Obstetrics and Gynaecology, 1st edn. London: RCOG Press, 2001: 59–69.

17.   Martin DC, Ling FW. Endometriosis and pain. Clin Obstet Gynecol 1999; 42: 664–86.

18.   Moen MH. Is mild endometriosis a disease? Why do women develop endometriosis and why is it diagnosed? Hum Reprod 1995; 10: 8–11.

19.   Smith A. Practical psychological approaches to women with pain. In MacLean AB, Stones RW, Thornton S, eds. Pain in Obstetrics and Gynaecology, 1st edn. London: RCOG Press, 2001: 70–86.

20.   Wood DP, Wiesner NG, Reiter RC. Psychogenic chronic pelvic pain: diagnosis and management. Clin Obstet Gynecol 1990; 33: 179–95.

21.   Collett BJ, Cordle C, Stewart C. Setting up a multidisciplinary clinic. Bailliere's Best Pract Res Clin Obstet Gynaecol 2000; 14: 541–56.

22.   Collett BJ, Cordle C, Stewart CR, Jagger C. A comparative study of women with chronic pelvic pain, chronic nonpelvic pain and those with no history of pain attending general practitioners. Br J Obstet Gynaecol 1998; 105: 87–92.

23.   Grace VM. Pitfalls of the medical paradigm in chronic pelvic pain. Bailliere's Best Pract Res Clin Obstet Gynaecol 2000; 14: 525–39.

24.   Baker PK. Musculoskeletal origins of chronic pelvic pain. Diagnosis and treatment. Obstet Gynecol Clin North Am 1993; 20: 719–42.

25.   Stones RW, Selfe SA. Doctors, women and pain. In MacLean AB, Stones RW, Thornton S, eds. Pain in Obstetrics and Gynaecology, 1st edn. London: RCOG Press, 2001: 152–63.

14

Hormonal therapy in chronic pelvic pain

William L Ledger

INTRODUCTION

'Hormonal therapy' for chronic cyclical pelvic pain describes a mixed bag of medical approaches used alone or in combination with analgesics and anti-inflammatory agents to try and reduce the impact of chronic pelvic pain on a patient's ability to function and enjoy a good quality of life. As discussed earlier in this book, individualization of management to meet patient needs is the cornerstone of a successful medical approach to chronic pelvic pain. Many patients will come with a complex history of previous surgical and medical interventions. Most will have a diagnosis of endometriosis of greater or lesser severity, but others will have been told that they have a 'normal pelvis' after laparoscopy, or present with any of a myriad other conditions that may cause pelvic pain.

The logic behind the use of hormonal therapy in chronic pelvic pain is to reduce or stop the ovarian cycle. Conditions such as endometriosis, which are believed to be driven by cyclical fluctuation in concentrations of estradiol (or other ovarian hormones), should then improve. Pain associated with endometriosis is thought to be the result of release of inflammatory mediators from endometriotic lesions in response to local changes in estradiol concentration. Pain related to deep lesions may be caused by infiltration or constriction of nerves or be secondary to adhesions[1], and may be less responsive to hormonal manipulation. The beneficial effects of removal of ovarian cyclicity on pelvic pain are likely to be temporary, with recurrence of symptoms as menses resume.

A number of hormonal therapies have been applied in chronic pelvic pain. These may be divided into oral contraceptive pills, progestogens, danazol, gonadotropin-releasing hormone (GnRH) analogs (agonists and antagonists) and newer aromatase inhibitors. The majority of research evidence concerns hormonal manipulation to manage chronic pelvic pain associated with endometriosis. Other causes of chronic pelvic pain have received less attention, and a medical approach to treatment is usually made after cross-reference with studies on patients with endometriosis. It seems reasonable to adopt this approach provided that the patient describes *cyclical* pelvic pain – this suggests a linkage with the ovarian cycle. Patients with constant or acyclic pain are less likely to benefit and other treatments should be used.

The management of pelvic pain associated with endometriosis has been outlined recently in guidelines issued by the Royal College of Obstetricians and Gynaecologists[2], with grades of evidence being allocated to individual recommendations. Details of the method of allocation can be gleaned from the guidelines themselves. The strength of evidence supporting individual recommendations will be given in this chapter to assist clinicians in making decisions in individual cases.

It is clear that endometriosis-associated pain can be managed effectively by medical therapy. Suppression of the ovarian cycle and induction of amenorrhea inactivates but does not remove local disease, and it is important for both doctor and patient to realize that symptoms recur after cessation of treatment in a proportion of patients. The various types of hormonal therapies used in endometriosis are believed to be of similar efficacy. Use in individual cases will be determined by tolerance of side-effects and reduction in health risks[2].

Given the frequent combination of chronic pelvic pain with infertility in endometriosis, it is important to recognize the lack of efficacy of medical therapy in the management of endometriosis-associated infertility. Use of medical therapy in this context will only delay pregnancy, and will not improve the chances of conception[2]. The only use for hormonal manipulation in this context may be to reduce pain symptoms whilst a patient is waiting to begin *in vitro* fertilization (IVF) treatment, and possibly to improve IVF outcome in patients with severe endometriosis[3].

THE COMBINED ORAL CONTRACEPTIVE PILL

The initial management of chronic pelvic pain in general practice frequently begins with introduction of a low-dose combined oral contraceptive pill, usually used continuously or tricyclically (i.e. 3 months of pills followed by a break to induce a menstrual bleed). More and better studies are needed to explore this approach systematically, as good evidence for efficacy and to provide guidance in choosing which pill, and for how long, is lacking[4]. One small randomized trial has compared cyclical administration of a low-dose combined oral contraceptive pill with a GnRH agonist for the treatment of non-menstrual pain and dyspareunia. Both approaches were found to be effective[4], and this evidence has been used to support use of the combined oral contraceptive pill as a first-line therapy. The Pill is relatively cheap and widely available. Its side-effect profile and relative and absolute contraindications are well understood. Importantly, young women may be happy to use the Pill to control pain and benefit from good-quality contraception. Again, this has to be discussed individually.

PROGESTOGENS

Continuous, high-dose administration of progestogens will inhibit ovulation and may also have a direct effect on endometriotic implants, leading to decidualization and eventual atrophy. Progestogens have been used for the treatment of endometriosis for a number of years but the most useful agents, doses and durations of treatment remain uncertain. Again, better-quality studies of adequate power are needed. The available evidence has recently been systematically reviewed[5]. There is support from randomized controlled trials for the use of both high-dose oral medroxyprogesterone acetate and depot medroxyprogesterone acetate (depo-Provera) for endometriosis-related pain. However, this therapy may lead to side-effects, including weight gain and breakthrough bleeding, headaches, nausea and, over long periods, loss of bone mineralization. In observational studies, lower doses of medroxyprogesterone acetate have been used with apparent success, an approach which may be helpful in reducing side-effects. Progestogens may be of use in the long-term management of endometriosis because of their low cost, safety and the availability of a 3-month depot preparation, improving patient compliance.

The Mirena levonorgestrel-releasing intrauterine device has been trialed for the management of endometriosis-related chronic pelvic pain in a pilot study[6], with apparent benefit. More recently, in another small non-randomized study of 34 women, the device was found to improve pain scores and reduce the severity of endometriotic lesions in women with mild or moderate disease, although again with problems of side-effects in some women[7].

DANAZOL

Danazol was first described for the treatment of menorrhagia in the late 1970s[8], and became widely used for the treatment of dysfunctional uterine bleeding and pelvic pain in the next decade. Danazol is a 19-nortestosterone-derived androgenic steroid which acts both centrally and locally to suppress steroidogenesis and induce endometrial atrophy. Its use in chronic pelvic pain has recently been systematically reviewed[9]. Danazol has been shown to improve pain and American Fertility Society scores in placebo-controlled trials. Although of confirmed efficacy, its use is limited by side-effects. Common side-effects are androgenic, including weight gain, acne, greasy skin, hirsutism and deepening of the voice, along with problems of breakthrough bleeding and limb tingling. Danazol may also have an adverse effect on serum lipids. In a small pilot study, danazol has been shown to suppress endometriosis at lower doses than those that suppress menstruation[10], a strategy that may allow more widespread use for patients who cannot tolerate side-effects at higher doses. Again, adequately powered randomized trials are needed in this area.

Gestrinone, a similar 19-nortestosterone, has been compared with danazol, a GnRH analog and placebo in randomized trials, with similar effects on pain scores but with fewer androgenic and hypoestrogenic side-effects than danazol and fewer hot flushes than with GnRH agonist[5]. There have not been comparative studies with progestogens. Gestrinone may represent a useful alternative to danazol for patients wishing to use this class of compounds. Issues such as cost and lack of long-term data should be taken into account.

GONADOTROPIN-RELEASING HORMONE ANALOGS

Analogs of GnRH resemble the structure of the native hypothalamic GnRH but carry peptide substitutions which increase their potency and half-life in the circulation. Analogs of GnRH with either agonist or antagonist properties have been developed[11]. The majority of clinical studies have been carried out with GnRH agonists, which have been used in gynecological practice since the early 1990s[12]. GnRH agonists initially stimulate the GnRH receptor, with release of follicle-stimulating hormone and luteinizing hormone, and a rise in the circulating concentration of estradiol. This 'flare' effect is followed within a few days by a long-term suppression of gonadotropin release, leading to 'pituitary down-regulation' and hypogonadism. Withdrawal of estradiol from the circulation removes its stimulatory effects from endometriotic deposits, resulting in shrinkage of lesions and reduction in pain. In contrast, the GnRH antagonists act directly on the pituitary GnRH receptors by competitive inhibition. They therefore have a more rapid onset of action than GnRH agonists. Whilst GnRH antagonists have been widely used for short-term pituitary suppression as part of IVF superovulation protocols, their use for longer-term therapy of chronic pelvic pain associated with endometriosis has been little explored[13]. GnRH antagonists may have specific and beneficial effects on endometriotic implants[14]. However, currently, treatment with GnRH antagonists requires a daily injection, while the agonists are available in 1- and 3-month depot formulations, with clear benefit to patients.

Use of GnRH agonists in endometriosis-associated chronic pelvic pain has recently been the subject of a Cochrane review[15]. This review concluded, on the basis of analysis of 26 randomized controlled trials, that the GnRH agonists are effective in the treatment of this condition. However, placebo-controlled trials of significant size have not been performed and the available studies concentrate almost exclusively on comparisons with other therapies. The effects on chronic pelvic pain appeared to be similar to those found with other medical treatments such as the combined oral contraceptive pill, danazol and gestrinone, but with different side-effect profiles. The GnRH agonists are non-androgenic, such that weight gain, acne, etc. do not appear commonly during treatment. However, the effects of estrogen withdrawal led to menopause-like side-effects that were common and distressing[15]. Most of the randomized controlled trials of GnRH agonists in chronic pelvic pain have been limited to 6 months' duration, and this length of time has been used to set the recommended maximum therapeutic exposure in the UK[16], with a recommendation that therapy should not be repeated. This recommendation is based on evidence of development of osteopenia due to hypoestrogenism during treatment[17,18]. The clinical response to GnRH agonist treatment has been found to be as great after 3 months of treatment as after 6 months[19], apart from the treatment of deep dyspareunia, for which 6 months of exposure was necessary to reach maximum benefit. However, whether treatment is used for 3 or 6 months, most women will experience recurrence in pain shortly after resumption of menses once treatment is discontinued. This is particularly the case for more severe forms of endometriosis[20], leading to a clinical need for strategies to allow longer-term use of the GnRH agonists.

A number of approaches have been used to try to remove the risk of developing significant osteopenia during longer-term exposure to GnRH agonists.

'Add-back' therapy with low-dose continuous estrogens has been recommended to prevent bone loss and minimize other side-effects. The 'estrogen threshold hypothesis'[21] suggests that there is a threshold for dosage with exogenous estrogens at which bone may be preserved without stimulation of endometriotic deposits, and has formed the basis for many studies of various add-back regimes[15,22,23]. Progestogens have also been used as add-back therapy with GnRH agonists[22]. More recently, longer-term studies have begun to suggest the possibility of extending the therapeutic window of use of GnRH agonists using add-back, although the studies are generally small sized[24,25]. For those who are unable to use hormonal add-back therapy, an alternative is to use bone-preserving agents such as the anti-absorptive bisphosphonates with regular monitoring of bone mineral density[26]. Again, research evidence in this area is limited and careful discussion is needed before embarking upon this approach.

AROMATASE INHIBITORS

Although GnRH agonist treatment with add-back is probably the most widely used medical treatment for significant degrees of endometriosis-related chronic pelvic pain in specialist practice, this may not be suitable for all patients and may require regular monitoring of bone mineral density. The drugs are also costly when used long term. The gold standard in medical therapy for endometriosis would be an oral medication which would successfully treat the symptoms and stop disease progression without the adverse side-effect profile of current orally active drugs such as danazol. One step closer to this gold standard may be the introduction of inhibitors of aromatase into gynecological practice. Aromatase synthesizes estrogens from androgenic precursors, and is found in endometriotic implants. Recent studies[27] have shown that aromatase inhibitors can induce regression of the implants with a reduction in pain. Since aromatase inhibitors have been used for some years to treat women with breast cancer, their safety and side-effect profiles are well known.

Ailawadi et al.[28] used the aromatase inhibitor letrozole in cases of endometriosis that had not responded well to other treatments. They studied 10 women with endometriosis-related pain who were given letrozole and a progestogen, norethindrone acetate, and vitamin D, to ameliorate bone loss. Treatment was for 6 months. At the end of this period, a repeat laparoscopy showed regression of the endometriosis implants and pain scores improved. Side-effects included hot flushes and sweats, although possibly less than those seen with GnRH agonists. Bone loss seemed to have been avoided by concurrent treatment with norethindrone and vitamin D. This pilot study should be followed by larger comparative randomized controlled trials against current therapies to establish the place of aromatase inhibitors in the treatment of chronic pelvic pain.

HORMONAL THERAPY AS AN ADJUNCT TO SURGERY

Although it may seem logical to induce pituitary down-regulation to shrink endometriotic lesions before surgery, there is no evidence that this is helpful, and it may complicate surgery by making it more difficult to identify the endometriotic deposits. Post-surgical treatment with GnRH agonists or combined oral contraceptive pills may help to delay the recurrence of chronic pelvic pain[29–31] although again, the best type and duration of treatment remain uncertain. If pregnancy is desired, it may be better to avoid postoperative medical treatment and encourage early resumption of regular intercourse.

HORMONAL THERAPY FOLLOWING BILATERAL OOPHORECTOMY FOR ENDOMETRIOSIS

One of the many clinical conundrums that bedevil this area of practice is that of when and how to use estrogen-based hormone replacement therapy (HRT) in young women who have had oophorectomy (usually with hysterectomy) as 'definitive' treatment for endometriosis. It is clear that exogenous estrogen therapy can reactivate endometriosis, with recurrence of pain and occasionally serious anatomical damage[32], although these cases are uncommon. Some form of protection against loss of bone mineral, and to minimize distressing systemic effects of estrogen lack after surgically induced menopause, is essential, particularly in this young group of patients. A small randomized trial has suggested that continuous combined HRT using tibolone may be preferable to the commonly used estrogen-only HRT prescribed after hysterectomy and bilateral oophorectomy[33]. Whether it is safe to start this treatment immediately following oophorectomy or after a delay of some months remains uncertain. Late recurrence of endometriosis resulting from hormone replacement has been reported.

CONCLUSIONS

Hormonal manipulation as a treatment for chronic pelvic pain is widely used. Given the usual prolonged course of the condition, a combined medical and surgical approach is usually adopted, with a move to another therapy if pain recurs. Although there is a reasonable evidence base for some of the medical treatments used, these are mainly studies funded by pharmaceutical companies that tend to focus on newer and more expensive products. Large gaps in knowledge remain, especially in the treatment of non-endometriotic pelvic pain.

REFERENCES

1.   Moore J, Kennedy S. Causes of chronic pelvic pain. Bailliere's Best Pract Res Clin Obstet Gynaecol 2000; 14: 389–402.

2.   Royal College of Obstetricians and Gynaecologists. The investigation and management of endometriosis. Royal College of Obstetricians and Gynaecologists, 2000, Guideline No 24.

3.   Marcus SF, Ledger WL. Efficacy and safety of long-acting GnRH agonists in in vitro fertilization and embryo transfer. Hum Fertil 2002; 4: 85–93.

4.   Moore J, Kennedy S, Prentice A. Modern combined oral contraceptives for pain associated with endometriosis. Cochrane Database Syst Rev 2000: CD001019.

5.   Prentice A, Deary AJ, Bland E. Progestogens and anti-progestogens for pain associated with endometriosis. Cochrane Database Syst Rev 2000: CD002122.

6.   Vercellini P, Aimi G, Panazza S, et al. A levonorgestrel-releasing intrauterine system for the treatment of dysmenorrhoea associated with endometriosis: a pilot study. Fertil Steril 1999; 72: 505–8.

7.   Lockhat FB, Emembolu JO, Konje JC. The evaluation of the effectiveness of an intrauterine-administered progestogen (levonorgestrel) in the symptomatic treatment of endometriosis and in the staging of the disease. Hum Reprod 2004; 19: 179–84.

8.   Chimbira TH, Cope E, Anderson AB, Bolton FG. The effect of danazol on menorrhagia, coagulation mechanisms, haematological indices and body weight. Br J Obstet Gynaecol 1979; 86: 46–50.

9. Selak V, Farquhar C, Prentice A, Singla A. Danazol for pelvic pain associated with endometriosis. Cochrane Database Syst Rev 2001: CD000068.

10. Vercellini P, Trespidi L, Panazza S, et al. Very low dose danazol for relief of endometriosis-associated pelvic pain: a pilot study. Fertil Steril 1994; 62: 1136–42.

11. Huirne JA, Lambalk CB. Gonadotropin-releasing-hormone-receptor antagonists. Lancet 2001; 358: 1793–1808.

12. Ledger WL, Thomas EJ, Browning D, et al. Suppression of gonadotrophin secretion does not reverse premature ovarian failure. Br J Obstet Gynaecol 1989; 96: 196–9.

13. Tarlatzis BC, Bili HN. Gonadotropin-releasing hormone antagonists: impact of IVF practice and potential non-assisted reproductive technology applications. Curr Opin Obstet Gynecol 2003; 15: 259–64.

14. Meresman GF, Bilotas MA, Lombardi E, et al. Effect of GnRH analogues on apoptosis and release of interleukin-1beta and vascular endothelial growth factor in endometrial cell cultures from patients with endometriosis. Hum Reprod 2003; 18: 1767–71.

15. Prentice A, Deary AJ, Goldbeck-Wood S, et al. Gonadotrophin-releasing hormone analogues for pain associated with endometriosis. Cochrane Database Syst Rev 2000: CD000346.

16. British National Formulary Number 36, 1998: 339.

17. Stevenson JC, Lees B, Gardner R, Shaw RW. A comparison of the skeletal effects of goserelin and danazol in premenopausal women with endometriosis. Horm Res 1989; 32 (Suppl 1): 161–3.

18. Compston JE, Yamaguchi K, Croucher PI, et al. The effects of gonadotrophin-releasing hormone agonists on iliac crest cancellous bone structure in women with endometriosis. Bone 1995; 16: 261–7.

19. Waller KG, Shaw RW. Gonadtrophin-hormone releasing hormone analogues for the treatment of endometriosis; long term follow up. Fertil Steril 1993; 59: 511–15.

20. Franke HR, van de Weijer PH, Pennings TM, van der Mooren MJ. Gonadotropin-releasing hormone agonist plus 'add-back' hormone replacement therapy for treatment of endometriosis: a prospective, randomized, placebo-controlled double-blind trial. Fertil Steril 2000; 74: 534–9.

21. Barbieri RL. Hormone treatment of endometriosis: the estrogen threshold hypothesis. Am J Obstet Gynecol 1992; 166: 740–5.

22. Hornstein MD, Surrey ES, Weisberg GW, Casino LA. Leuprolide acetate depot and hormonal add-back in endometriosis: a 12-month study. Leupron Add-Back Study Group. Obstet Gynecol 1998; 91: 16–24.

23. Kiesel L, Schweppe KW, Sillem M, Siebzehnrubl E. Should add-back therapy for endometriosis be deferred for optimal results? Br J Obstet Gynaecol 1996; 103 (Suppl 14): 15–17.

24. Pierce SJ, Gazvani MR, Farquharson RG. Long-term use of gonadotrophin-releasing hormone analogues and hormone replacement therapy in the management of endometriosis: a randomized trial with a 6-year follow-up. Fertil Steril 2000; 74: 964–8.

25. Surrey ES, Silverberg KM, Surrey MW, Schoolcraft WB. Effect of prolonged gonadotrophin-releasing hormone agonist therapy on the outcome of in vitro fertilization-embryo transfer in patients with endometriosis. Fertil Steril 2002; 78: 699–704.

26. Mukherjee T, Baraad D, Turk R, Freeman R. A randomized placebo-controlled study on the effect of cyclic intermittent etidronate therapy on the bone mineral density changes associated with six months of gonadotrophin-releasing hormone agonist treatment. Am J Obstet Gynecol 1996; 175: 105–9.

27. Ebert AD, Bartley J, David M. Aromatase inhibitors and cyclooxygenase-2 (COX-2) inhibitors in endometriosis: new questions – old answers? Eur J Obstet Gynecol Reprod Biol 2005 Sep 9, (Epub ahead of print).

28. Ailawadi RK, Jobanputra S, Kataria M, et al. Treatment of endometriosis and chronic pelvic pain with letrozole and norethindrone acetate: a pilot study. Fertil Steril 2004; 81: 290–6.

29. Hornstein MD, Hemmings R, Yuzpe AA, Heinrichs WL. Use of nafarelin versus placebo after reductive laparoscopic surgery for endometriosis. Fertil Steril 1997; 68: 860–4.

30. Vercellini P, Crosignani PG, Fadini R, et al. A gonadotrophin-releasing hormone agonist compared with expectant management after conservative surgery for symptomatic endometriosis. Br J Obstet Gynaecol 1999; 106: 672–7.

31. Muzii M, Marana R, Caruana P, et al. Postoperative administration of monophasic combined oral contraceptives after laparoscopic treatment of ovarian endometriomas: a prospective, randomised trial. Am J Obstet Gynecol 2000; 183: 588–92.

32. Matorras R, Elorriaga MA, Pijoan JI, et al. Recurrence of endometriosis in women with bilateral adnexectomy (with or without total hysterectomy) who received hormone replacement therapy. Fertil Steril 2002; 77: 303–8.

33. Fedele L, Bianchi S, Rafaelli R, Zanconato G. Comparison of transdermal estradiol and tibolone for the treatment of oophorectomised women with deep residual endometriosis. Maturitas 1999; 32: 189–93.

Index

CPP = chronic pelvic pain; tables and diagrams are denoted by **bold** page numbers